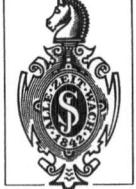

Motor Behavior

Programming, Control, and Acquisition

Edited by
H. Heuer, U. Kleinbeck
and K.-H. Schmidt

With Contributions by
J. Annett, W. D. A. Beggs, C. H. M. Brunia
S. A. V. M. Haagh, P. A. Hancock, C. I. Howarth
B. J. Leikind, K. M. Newell, D. A. Rosenbaum
J. G. M. Scheirs, R. A. Schmidt, D. E. Sherwood
H. N. Zelaznik

With 80 Figures

Springer-Verlag
Berlin Heidelberg New York Tokyo

Professor Dr. HERBERT HEUER
Abteilung für Psychologie der Universität Bielefeld,
Postfach 86 40, 4800 Bielefeld, FRG

Professor Dr. UWE KLEINBECK
Bergische Universität-Gesamthochschule Wuppertal,
Fach Psychologie, Gaußstraße 20,
5600 Wuppertal, FRG

Dipl.-Psych. KLAUS-HELMUT SCHMIDT
Institut für Arbeitsphysiologie an der Universität Dortmund,
Ardeystraße 67,
4600 Dortmund, FRG

ISBN-13:978-3-642-69751-7   e-ISBN-13:978-3-642-69749-4
DOI: 10.1007/978-3-642-69749-4

Library of Congress Cataloging in Publication Data. Main entry under title: Motor behavior. Bibliography: p.   Includes indexes. 1. Motor ability. 2. Perceptual-motor processes. 3. Self-control. 4. Movement, Psychology of. I. Heuer, H.(Herbert), 1948– . II. Kleinbeck, Uwe. III. Schmidt, K.-H. (Klaus-Helmut), 1952– . IV. Annett, John. BF295.M65   1985   152.3   85-12672

2126/3130-543210

Preface

In recent years there has been steadily increasing interest in motor behavior and a growing awareness that a person not only has to know *what* to do in a particular situation, but also *how* to do it. The question of how actions are performed is of central concern in the area of motor control. This volume provides an advanced-level treatment of some of the main issues.

Experiments concerned with basic processes of motor control typically examine very simple movements. At first glance these tasks appear to be far removed from real-world tasks, but it should be kept in mind that they are not studied for their own sake. One of the main reasons for using them is the well-recognized, but sometimes questioned, scientific principle that basic laws may be discovered more easily in simple situations than in complex situations. Another reason is that the simple tasks studied constitute building blocks of more complex tasks. For example, some complex skills can be considered as consisting of sequences of aimed movements, although, as no one would doubt, knowing everything about these individual movements does not mean knowing everything about, for example, typing.

The first two chapters of the present volume focus on behavioral and physiological studies of programming and preparation of movements. In the first chapter D. Rosenbaum introduces the concept of a motor program that is set up in advance of the overt movement. He then discusses the major questions that arise with respect to such programs and the current answers based on behavioral data. Finally, he sets forth a general framework for conceptualizing the programming of movements.

A quite different approach to the preparatory processes that precede execution of a movement is presented in the chapter by C. H. M. Brunia, S. A. V. M. Haagh, and J. G. M. Scheirs. By means of physiological recording techniques it is possible to trace preparatory processes at the cortical and spinal levels. One of the main questions addressed is the role of different brain structures in motor preparation. To the extent that functions of different brain structures are known, this approach also helps to answer questions about which functions are involved in preparing a movement. One of the challenging tasks of the future is to tie together the two different approaches to motor preparation that are represented by these first two chapters.

Chapters 3 to 5 focus on the control of movements, in particular on the control of aiming movements. A common theme is the relationship between speed and accuracy. R. A. Schmidt, D. E. Sherwood, H. N. Zelaznik, and B. J. Leikind begin this section with an open-loop interpretation of this relationship based on the concept of a generalized motor program. At least in very fast movements, considerable support can be found for the underlying principles of this theory, but the authors also discuss the difficulties and unsolved problems.

C. I. Howarth and W. D. A. Beggs approach the relationship between speed and accuracy from a quite different viewpoint, focussing on movements in which there is sufficient time for closed-loop control. Accuracy of movement is related to temporal delays in the processing of visual feedback and to the inaccuracy of spatial information. Although the open-loop and closed-loop approaches to the problem of speed-accuracy tradeoff might appear to be contradictory, they are certainly not; they concentrate on different relevant aspects. It should in principle be possible to unify the two theories, although this has not yet been done. It is by now widely recognized that closed-loop control and open-loop control are not mutually exclusive, and that the problem is to identify the principles by which these two modes of control can be combined.

While the first two chapters on the control of movements elaborate on particular theories, the next chapter, by P. A. Hancock and K. M. Newell, takes a more comprehensive, descriptive approach to the problem of speed and accuracy. From a review of the classical data a general description of the relationship between speed, amplitude, duration, and different measures of error is developed; this is then extended to temporal accuracy. In the process the shortcomings of various theories are noted. The general description of spatial and temporal error functions constitutes a challenge for any comprehensive theory of the control of aiming movements.

The final chapter of the book focusses on long-term changes in motor control. J. Annett explicitly omits traditional topics in the area of motor learning and concentrates instead on the current major problems which link this area to other fields of experimental psychology. First, he elaborates on the fact that motor learning is not a problem at the periphery of psychology, but rather is strongly dependent on various purely mental processes like imagery and verbal coding. This view challenges the classical view that cognitive processes are important only in the first stages of motor learning. In the second part of the chapter some of the recent ideas on why practice helps to improve performance are reviewed. The reader may note that some of these ideas are in fact new versions of very old ones, dating back to the turn of the century, a time when the field of learning was not yet dominated by the notion of reinforcement and related concepts.

The chapters in this volume were given impetus by the symposium "Psychology of Motor Behavior," held in Dortmund in March 1983. We acknowledge the financial support of the *Deutsche Forschungsgemeinschaft* and express our gratitude to the authors and reviewers.

Bielefeld, Wuppertal,   HERBERT HEUER
and Dortmund, 1985   UWE KLEINBECK
                                                                   KLAUS-HELMUT SCHMIDT

Contents

List of Contributors

J. ANNETT, Department of Psychology, University of Warwick, Coventry CV4 7AL, United Kingdom

W. D. A. BEGGS, Department of Psychology, University of Nottingham, Nottingham NG7 2RD, United Kingdom

C. H. M. BRUNIA, Department of Psychology, Physiological Psychology Section, Tilburg University, 5000 LE Tilburg, The Netherlands

S. A. V. M. HAAGH, Department of Psychology, Physiological Psychology Section, Tilburg University, 5000 LE Tilburg, The Netherlands

P. A. HANCOCK, Department of Safety Science, Institute of Safety and Systems Management, University of Southern California, Los Angeles, CA 90089, USA

C. I. HOWARTH, Department of Psychology, University of Nottingham, Nottingham NG7 2RD, United Kingdom

B. J. LEIKIND, Department of Physics, University of California, Los Angeles, CA 90024, USA

K. M. NEWELL, Motor Behavior Laboratory, University of Illinois at Urbana-Champaign, IL 61820, USA

D. A. ROSENBAUM, School of Communications and Cognitive Science, Hampshire College, Amherst, MA 01002, USA

J. G. M. SCHEIRS, Department of Psychology, Physiological Psychology Section, Tilburg University, 5000 LE Tilburg, The Netherlands

R. A. SCHMIDT, Motor Control Laboratory, Department of Kinesiology, University of California, Los Angeles, CA 90024, USA

D. E. SHERWOOD, Motor Control Laboratory, Department of Kinesiology, University of California, Los Angeles, CA 90024, USA

H. N. ZELAZNIK, Department of Physical Education, Health, and Recreation Studies, Purdue University, West Lafayette, IN 47907, USA

Motor Programming:
A Review and Scheduling Theory

D. A. ROSENBAUM

Contents

Introduction

The problem of the control of action has long occupied the interests of philosophers and physiologists. For philosophers, the problem historically has concerned the nature of the will: Are people free to choose their own actions? Are they different from animals in this respect? For physiologists, the problem has concerned mechanism: How are the neuromuscular activities of the body coordinated in such a way that skillful, or not such skillful, movements occur?

For psychologists, the problem of action control lies somewhere between these two. Whenever a "voluntary" movement is produced, there seems to be an issuance of the will. Although you could at this moment be watching a movie or riding a bicycle, you have chosen instead, presumably freely, to read this chapter. At a more mundane level of decision-making you have also decided to assume some posture while reading, this chapter, to bring your eyes to where they are at this moment, and so on. For the psychologist, perhaps the most intriguing question underlying the study of action control is how intentions are translated into actions. For me personally, one reason why I have chosen to study motor programming is to gain access to the will itself.

To begin the discussion of motor programming from the standpoint of the will is, on some investigator's accounts, to place the ghost before the machine. Why, they would ask, should one impute to the organism something as elusive as the will in attempting to explain how animals navigate through a well-structured optical environment, how primates carry out coordinated reaching movements, how humans move their lips, and so on? The answer depends on what one is trying to explain. If one is after a totally mechanistic account of the control of physical behavior, then starting with the will may not be the most desirable starting point. As Turvey and others have argued (Kelso, Tuller, and Harris 1983; Pew 1984; Turvey 1977), in starting "intentionally" one runs the risk of placing too much theoretical baggage in the mind, where it is relatively inaccessible, and not enough in the peripheral motor system, where direct observation and tests of known mechanical laws are more easily achieved.

This is a sensible approach to science. One would like whenever possible to be able to explain things in terms that are familiar and well established, leaving only those things that cannot be explained to new domains of discovery. Plainly, if the knee jerk can be understood in terms of identifiable myoelectric circuits, then little is gained, and indeed something may be lost, by bringing in unneeded intentions.

Why then should one take as one's object of study the question of how intentions are translated into actions, that being the question at the heart of the study of motor programming? For me there are two principal answers. One is that a commonsense view of the production of movement must assume that except for "reflex" motions such as the knee jerk, actions begin with some *decision* about what is to be achieved. How else could one explain the enormous range of actions and qualities of performance that occur in the same stimulus conditions? The other reason for acknowledging the importance of intentions is that constructs such as plans and intentions no longer have the questionable epistemological status they did before the emergence of cognitive psychology. It is now clear that people engage in covert mental activity that allows for the constructive elaboration of experience, both past and future. To deny the reality of such activity in the domain of motor performance would be to backtrack significantly in our investigation of the control of behavior (Powers 1973). By the same token, granting the reality and importance of intention leads one to reject the idea that intention can merely be regarded as what is left over after biomechanical analyses have explained all they can.

In this chapter I review the evidence that has led to the postulation of motor programs. Then I turn to the major questions that have occupied and continue to occupy students of motor programming. In the final portions of the chapter I introduce a theoretical framework for studying motor programming, considering data that support the framework and pointing to areas in which the framework needs to be extended or refined.

Evidence and Definitions

Two principal lines of evidence make it clear that orderly patterns of nervous activity precede and allow for the production of skilled voluntary movements. Insofar as this nervous activity is related to the retrieval and formation of representations governing the control of forthcoming movements, these lines of evidence show that motor programs are real rather than imagined entities.

Independence From Sensory Feedback

One of the main sources of evidence for motor programs is that skillful movement is often possible when feedback is disrupted. For example, Lashley (1917) reported that a patient with a gunshot wound that eliminated sensation could reproduce movements accurately. In a later, more controlled study, Taub and Berman (1968) showed that monkeys that were surgically deprived of normal proprioceptive feedback could still carry out skillful reaching and locomotor movements. Similar capacities have been reported by other investigators working with a wide range of species (for reviews see Keele 1968; Evarts, Bizzi, Burke, De-Long, and Thach 1971).

It is important to appreciate the logical implications of this general result. One could imagine a motor control system in which the sensory feedback from one movement triggers the next movement to be carried out. Indeed, during the first half of the twentieth century behaviorists took this possibility so seriously that they made a theoretical commitment to the idea of "reflex chaining," and eschewed any discussion of unobservable structures such as motor programs. The repudiation of reflex chain theory is so fundamental to the concept of the motor program that Keele (1968) based his definition of the motor program on it. The motor program, Keele wrote, is "a set of movement instructions that are structured before a movement sequence begins, and that allows the entire sequence to be carried out uninfluenced by peripheral feedback" (p. 387). Similarly, Schmidt (in Kelso, 1982) defined the motor program as "an abstract memory structure prepared before the movement which, when executed, results in movement without the involvement of feedback requiring a correction for an error in selection" (p. 291).

Besides the demonstration that skilled performance resists feedback removal, another outcome which suggests that sensory feedback need not play a determining role in movement selection is that delays between successive movements seem to be too short to allow for sensory feedback to determine what movement should be performed after another movement has been completed. Lashley (1951) made this argument in connection with piano playing. He was struck by the fact that accomplished pianists can play sequences of keystrokes at rates exceeding 10/s. Since Lashley thought it takes more than 1/10 s to process sensory feedback, he questioned the plausibility of reflex chain theory. Lashley's argument is compromised by the fact that sensory signals have recently been found to reach the cortex in 10 msec or less (see Adams 1976). Moreover, his argument is open to the criticism that even if one movement is not triggered by feedback from the immediately preceding movement, it could still be triggered by movements occurring earlier. Thus a "movement speed" argument carries less weight for motor programs than does the "feedback disruption" argument presented earlier.

Some caution is needed in thinking of motor programs exclusively in terms of their allowance for ballistic control. Some investigators who have found that feedback *can* influence motor performance have concluded that motor programs do not exist. This conclusion is reasonable given Keele's and Schmidt's definitions. However, a broader conception of motor programs allows for the possibility that they permit different courses of action depending on exigencies of actual performance. An example that captures this type of control comes from a study by Forssberg, Grillner, and Rossignol (1975). These investigators applied a tactile stimulus to the paw of a cat walking on a treadmill. When the stimulus was applied at the start of the swing phase of gait the cat flexed its leg more than usual. When the same stimulus was applied during the stance phase, the cat extended its leg more than usual. Thus, the same stimulus – or what is *assumed* to be the same stimulus – had dramatically different effects on performance depending on when it occurred. Presumably, this result came about because of some central change that occurred during the gait cycle. The finding that the same sensory feedback can give rise to different motor reactions depending on the context in which the reactions occur is a third source of evidence against the reflex chain theory.

If it is allowed that motor programs provide for contextually dependent reactions to feedback, then they can be likened to computer programs that produce different outputs depending on the values supplied to the functions they employ. Recently, several authors have defined motor programs without specific reference to ballistic control. For example, van Galen and Teulings (1983) defined the motor program as simply "the central representation of an ordered sequence of movement elements" (p. 10), and Shaffer (1982) adopted the definition "a set of grammatical representations of intended action constructed, by a control system, as a hierarchy of abstractions, terminating in motor output" (p. 110).

Anticipatory Effects

Although the demonstration of independence from feedback has been vital for the postulation of motor programs, anticipatory effects have been no less important. A wide range of anticipatory phenomena have been studied, the major classes of which will be discussed below. All of these phenomena show systematic changes in behavior (or some physiological concomitant of behavior) that correlates with some aspect of forthcoming behavior. The presence of such well-defined anticipatory effects implies that some representation for the forthcoming action exists within the nervous system.

Perhaps the most dramatic kinds of anticipatory effects are those in which overt behavior changes depending on the movements that are about to be performed. Coarticulation effects in speech comprise one class of such effects (Kent and Minifie 1977), as do kinematic adjustments in the early phases of manual reaching movements depending on how those movements will end (cf. Hinton, 1984).

More subtle anticipatory effects are observed with physiological, perceptual, and chronometric measurements. Among the physiological indices of forthcoming movements are changes in reflex excitability (see Brunia, this volume) and brain activity (e.g., Deecke, Grozinger, and Kornhuber 1976; Evarts 1984; Requin, Lecas, and Bonnet 1984). Perceptual changes that presage motor activity include saccadic suppression, which begins even before the eyes start to saccade (Volkmann, Schick, and Riggs, 1969), and blink suppression, which begins even before the onset of eyeblinks (Volkmann, Riggs, and Moore 1980). These results suggest that internal perceptual changes occur prior to eye movements, consistent with the programming position.

Chronometric analyses also provide dramatic evidence for anticipatory effects in motor performance. For example, Shaffer (1976), in studying the timing of keystrokes in typing, observed that latencies of the first few keystrokes in a word depended on identities of later keystrokes. In reaction-time experiments, where subjects are instructed to begin responding as quickly as possible after the appearance of a signal, the time to begin responding has been found to depend on characteristics of the responses to be performed. For example, Henry and Rogers (1980) and Sternberg, Monsell, Knoll, and Wright (1978) found that the reaction time to produce the first of a series of responses increased with the length of the series. Such an effect would not be expected if a program for the entire sequence had not been prepared in advance.

Programs Versus Plans

Having mentioned some of the main lines of evidence for motor programs and the principal definitions that have been offered for them, it is important to clarify the distinction between programs and plans. Generally, the term program is reserved for lower-level forms of preparation. Thus, it would be inappropriate to say that one is developing a motor program for a trip to Germany but it would be appropriate to say that one is developing a plan for such a trip. Programmed spans of activity are considerably shorter than planned spans of activity, and programs, in contrast to plans, are thought to lead directly to motor activity. Finally, planning may have a conscious component, but programming is generally considered to occur outside conscious awareness.

Issues in the Study of Motor Programs

In view of the convergent evidence for motor programs, more detailed questions
arise about their characteristics and evolution. Six principal questions can be
posed: (1) How are motor programs structured? (2) What are their parameters and units? (3) How do they incorporate biomechanical constraints? (4) How
are they constructed in real time prior to their execution? (5) How are they
stored? (6) How are they learned? In the discussion below I consider each of
these questions in turn.

Structure

Although the execution of successive movements by a skilled performer may appear, for all intents and purposes. as a smooth stream of behavior, it is not obvious that the motor program guiding production of that behavioral sequence is a
linear string of instructions. Instead, it may be a more complex, nested set of instructions whose detailed structure can only be inferred through the examination
of response timing or subtle performance errors.

  Although many psychologists have long suspected that the control of motor
behavior is hierarchical (e.g., Miller, Galanter, and Pribram 1960), strong evidence for this hypothesis appeared only recently. In one study (Rosenbaum,
Kenny, and Derr 1983) subjects produced memorized sequences of finger responses such as those used in piano-playing. The sequences studied were purposely chosen because they are easily organized in a hierarchical fashion. The
reasoning was that if any sequences are hierarchically controlled these should be.

  As seen in Fig. 1, the time to perform each response after the immediately
preceding response depended on its serial position. The data are most easily interpreted within the framework of hierarchical control, as seen in Fig. 2. If control passes through a hierarchy according to the rules of a tree-traversal process
and if the time to move from one node to the next is assumed to take a finite and
measurable amount of time, then the larger the number of nodes to be traversed
between successive responses the longer the corresponding interresponse time
should be. Figure 3 shows that this prediction was supported. When interresponse time was plotted against number of nodes traversed, a linear function
emerged. Other studies have reported qualitatively similar results (Povel and Collard 1982; Schneider and Fisk 1983).

  The tree-traversal conception of response production also accounts for data
from reaction-time experiments reported by Sternberg et al. (1978). These investigators recorded the latency of response sequences consisting of variable numbers of typewriting keystrokes or, in other conditions, spoken words. Subjects
were told in advance what responses would have to be produced and were instructed to minimize the time between detection of the reaction signal and completion of the required sequence. Three main results were obtained. First, the
time to produce the first response in the sequence increased with the total length

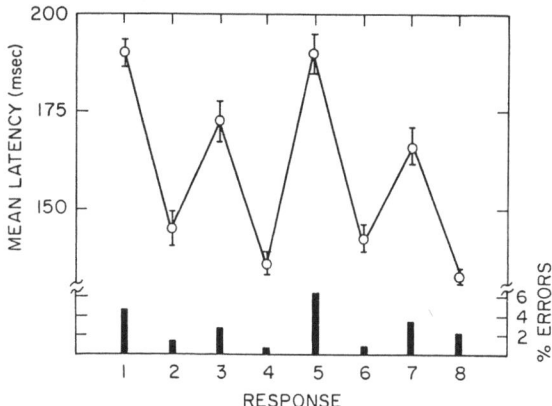

Fig. 1. Mean latencies of responses 1–8 in the rapid finger sequencies such as IiIiMmMm, where I and i denote right and left index fingers, respectively, M and m denote right and left middle fingers, respectively. (From "Hierarchical control of rapid movement sequences" by Rosenbaum, Kenny, and Derr, *Journal of Experimental Psychology: Human Perception and Performance,* 1983, 86–102. Copyright 1983 by the American Psychological Association. Reprinted by permission of the publisher)

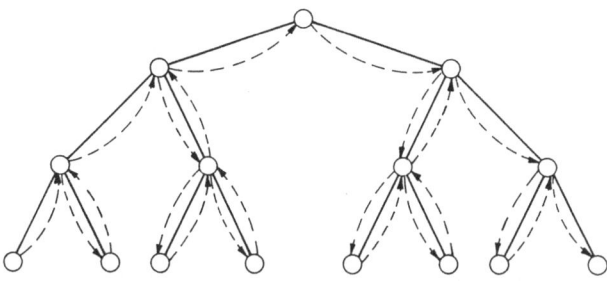

Fig. 2. Tree-traversal process hypothesized to underlie control of rapid finger sequences. (From "Hierarchical control of rapid movement sequences" by Rosenbaum, Kenny, and Derr, *Journal of Experimental Psychology: Human Perception and Performance,* 1983, *9,* 86–102. Copyright 1983 by the American Psychological Association. Reprinted by permission of the publisher)

of the sequence. Second, the mean time between responses within the sequences also increased with sequence length, the rate of increase often being approximately the same as the rate of increase for the latency of the first response. Third, latencies of individual responses depended on their serial positions such that responses in the middle of the sequence had longer latencies than responses near the beginning or end.

Sternberg et al. accounted for these results with a *buffer search* model. According to the model, a program for the entire forthcoming response sequence is

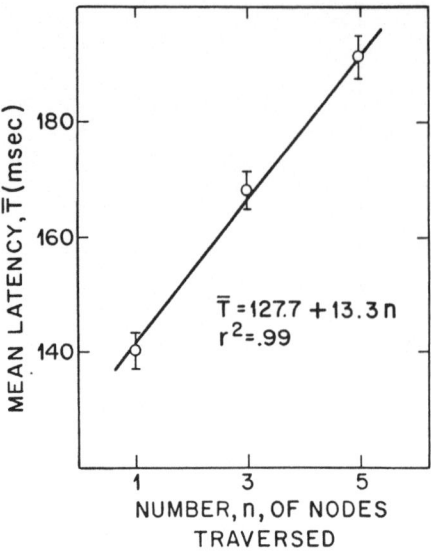

Fig. 3. Mean latency as a function of number of hypothesized tree-traversal steps. (From "Hierarchical control of rapid movement sequences" by Rosenbaum, Kenny, and Derr, *Journal of Experimental Psychology: Human Perception and Performance, 1983, 9, 86–102.* Copyright 1983 by the American Psychological Association. Reprint by permission of the publisher)

loaded into a buffer which must be searched prior to the performance of each response in order to locate the subprogram for that response. Sternberg et al. claimed that as the number of to-be-searched subprograms increased, the mean time to locate the required subprogram also increased, giving the first and second results described above. As for the third result, concerning serial position effects, Sternberg et al. (p. 147) confessed that their model did not uniquely predict the shape of the serial position function they obtained.

The three-traversal model proposed by Rosenbaum et al. (1983) predicts the serial position effects of Sternberg et al., as well as their initial latency and interresponse time results. As was seen in Fig. 2, a distinct pattern of interresponse times was obtained over serial positions in the finger-tapping study of Rosenbaum et al., and, as was seen in Fig. 3, a tree-traversal model accounted for those data quite well. If one counts the number of nodes traversed between the first response and second, between the second response and third, and so on, the numbers are 2, 4, 2, 6, 2, 4, and 2. Thus the largest number of nodes traversed occupies the middle position, which is consistent with the general trend observed by Sternberg et al., and the mean number of steps before each noninitial response is $(2+4+2+6+2+4+2)/7 = 3.14$. As seen in Table 1, the three-traversal model predicts that the mean number of steps for sequences consisting of

Table 1. Mean number of steps predicted by the tree-traversal model for responses 1–6 in sequences of length 2–6 [a]

Length	Response						Mean (2–6)
	1	2	3	4	5	6	
2	2.0	2.0					2.0
3	2.5	2.5	2.5				2.5
4	3.0	2.0	4.0	2.0			2.7
5	3.3	2.3	3.5	3.5	2.3		2.9
6	3.5	2.3	3.5	3.6	3.5	2.3	3.0

[a] The number of steps for response 1 was derived by starting at the top node of the tree and proceeding downward to the terminal node corresponding to the first response. The latency of each response is assumed to be a linear function of the number of immediately preceding tree-traversal steps, with the intercept of the linear function being higher for response 1 than for noninitial responses due to the extra time needed for processing of the reaction signal.

fewer than eight responses should increase with the number of responses, as Sternberg et al. found. Moreover, the model predicts that interresponse times should always be longer in the middle of the sequence than at the ends. (These theoretical data were obtained by drawing all possible multi-tiered hierarchies for sequences of 2, 3, 5, and 6 responses, counting the number of nodes to be traversed in reaching each response after the immediately preceding response, and averaging over the total number of hierarchies for each sequence length. For sequences with four responses, only a perfect binary tree was used.)

It should be noted that there is still some debate about the notion that motor programs are hierarchically structured. Klein (1983), for example, suggested that the timing results of Rosenbaum et al. could be accounted for with a non-hierarchical logogen model, although major difficulties with this position were pointed out by Rosenbaum (1983 b). Salthouse (1984) recently reported data suggesting that in transcription typing there is no chunking of successive keystrokes into higher-level units. He found, for example, that the time for the first keystroke in a word did *not* increase with the number of keystrokes in the word. It may be that the structuring of motor programs depends to some extent on the nature of the input signal to the motor system. Continuously available text may not require the same degree of chunking as text that is memorized.

Parameters and Units

Intimately related to the question of how motor programs are structured is the question of what the units and parameters of motor programs are. One way of learning about the units of motor programs is to identify the variables that affect the reaction time for a forthcoming movement sequence. Those variables that consistently influence reaction time can be assumed to relate in some direct way to the units of motor programs. Sternberg et al. adopted this logic in their study of rapid speech production. They found that speech reaction time increased with the number of stress units to be produced, suggesting that stress units are the basic units for speech motor programs. A similar approach was taken by Teulings, Thomassen, and van Galen (1983) in a study of handwriting. Their subjects produced pairs of cursive letters in simple and choice reaction-time conditions. In the choice reaction-time condition there was no benefit from congruence of *strokes* between the two letters within the pair, although benefits did accrue from congruence of *letters* within the pair. Teulings et al. argued that letters rather than strokes are the basic units of handwriting, a claim they acknowledged to be at odds with previous work on the control of handwriting. The uncertainty about the basic units of handwriting is representative of the uncertainty surrounding basic units in other performance domains (see Kerr 1978; Marteniuk and MacKenzie, 1980).

Whereas questions about basic units are easily raised in the domain of serially produced "discrete" movements, comparable questions about the basic *parameters* of control arise in connection with "continuous" movements. One can get a feeling for this issue by considering manual reaching movements. When the hand is moved to a particular location the motion can be described in terms of the direction pursued, the distance covered, the peak velocity achieved, the torques acting on the joints, and so on. Clearly, there is some redundancy among these alternative descriptions, which suggests that within the motor system as well only some of the parameters may actually be employed. Discovering which parameters are used is one of the major challenges of research on motor programming. In the case of aimed hand movements, there is evidence that final *location* rather than distance and direction may be the relevant programming parameter (Polit and Bizzi 1978). Likewise, saccadic eye movements appear to be programmed with respect to target location (Guthrie, Porter, and Sparks 1983), and target location has also been posited as the critical programming parameter in articulatory control (MacNeilage 1970).

Polit and Bizzi (1978) argued for location-setting for arm movements based on the remarkable ability of deafferented monkeys to make accurate pointing movements without the aid of visual feedback, even after mechanical perturbations were momentarily applied to the limb. Guthrie et al. (1983) concluded that eye movements are programmed with respect to final location based on an experiment in which monkeys were rewarded for making eye movements to a briefly illuminated spot of light. Just after the spot was presented but before the eyes began to move, an electrical pulse was delivered to the superior colliculus. The pulse caused a slight involuntary movement of the eyes, but not toward the target. Nevertheless, the eyes reached the target appropriately despite the absence of feedback. Thus, the monkeys in this experiment made accurate eye movements following brief electrical perturbations, just as the monkeys of Bizzi et al. made accurate arm movements following brief mechanical perturbations. If the eye and arm movements had been programmed with respect to direction and distance, the final locations achieved would have been systematically incorrect. The ability to compensate in this fashion can be taken as evidence for the mass-spring model of limb movement control (Fel'dman 1966). Interestingly, Mac-Neilage's (1970) proposal for location programming in articulation is based on feedforward-feedback considerations involving the muscle spindles (Merton 1972).

Physiological evidence is not the only kind that has been used to infer the underlying parameters of motor programming. Observations of the kinematics of movement have also served this purpose. The principal approach has been to identify aspects of movements that can be varied independently of one another and then to argue that those aspects are at least representative of underlying control parameters (see Rosenbaum 1980, p. 453). In one of the most detailed and successful applications of this approach, Meyer, Smith, and Wright (1982) reviewed data showing that force and time are independent control parameters for limb movements. The independence of these two parameters will prove important in the theorizing to be presented later in this chapter.

Biomechanical Constraints

The discussion of motor programming cannot proceed without attention to the properties of the neuromotor system itself. Several authors have criticized motor programming research for not paying enough attention to these factors. Witness the following quotation from Kelso et al. (1983):

> The claim that programs can be developed to model the human mind is vacuous: Without the incorporation of constraints, one program may be as good as any other, and none may have anything to do with how real biological systems work ... The motor program notion, for example, is a description of an act – specified in terms of contractions of muscles – that is too powerful because it can describe acts that could never be performed by an actor. Theoretically, the motor program is as viable for unorganized convulsions as it is for coordinated movement. (p. 141)

Kelso et al. make an important point here, although I disagree with the way they have represented the motor program concept or the efforts of those seeking to delineate its properties. It is certainly too restrictive to say that "the motor program is a description of an act ... specified in terms of contractions of muscles." Much discussion among students of motor programming has centered on the question of whether muscle contractions are the primitive elements of motor programs, and the prevailing view is that they are not (Klapp 1977). Second, it is not really fair to say that because the concept of the motor program is as yet relatively unconstrained it should be viewed as a concept of limited utility. If one were to adopt this point of view generally in the discussion of hypothetical constructs, one would never be able to posit the existence of anything whose properties were not yet fully understood. One of the central objectives of students of motor programming is to determine what the bounds of motor programs are. Thus, an important aim of motor programming research is to identify the properties of motor programs that allow for the performance of some actions but not others. In this sense, the study of motor programming is similar to the study of linguistics. Just as there may be a finite number of rules that limit the set of allowable sentences in a language, so too may there be a limited number of rules, incorporated into motor programs, which restrict the set of movements that can be carried out.

Construction

Whereas the preceding discussion was concerned with the *structure* of motor programs, it is no less important to consider how motor programs are set up in real time. What, in other words, is the nature of the motor programming *process?* In approaching this question, it is useful to distinguish among three general models (see Rosenbaum 1983 b).

According to one, there are distinct, prepackaged programs for every movement sequence that an individual can possibly perform. This is a straw man, of course, because the infinite variety of movements precludes the possibility that every movement has its own defining program. Yet the model deserves mention because it suggests one possible view of the motor programming process, namely, that motor programming consists of *retrieving* prepackaged programs.

Another extreme position is that there are no prepackaged programs at all, only raw building blocks out of which programs are put together on a "demand" basis. In this scenario, motor programming consists of selecting and assembling these raw building blocks.

A third model is intermediate between these two. It says that there are prepackaged programs whose exact form at execution time is determined by the variables input to them just beforehand. Programming here consists of selecting holistic movement instructions (i.e., prepackaged motor programs) and selecting and inputting abstract motor variables to the programs that are selected.

Of the three models mentioned above, the one that is most clearly supported by existing data is the third one. The most obvious reason to favor this alternative is that skills generalize: Someone who plays the violin adroitly can easily learn to play the viola, for example. If motor programs were only temporarily joined motor variables, it would be hard to see how the acquisition of viola playing would benefit from prior experience with the violin, and if stored motor programs were represented in an entirely holistic fashion, it is hard to see how the skill associated with violin playing could transfer to the viola.

Adopting the view that motor programs are both stored holistically and "filled in" or modified through the assignment of values to them means that the process of motor programming consists of two distinct processes. One, as was said earlier, is selecting appropriate programs; the other is selecting and supplying appropriate values to the programs that have been selected. Given this bipartite view, it is important to identify the subprocess in which the parameters and units of motor programs come into play. Thus, if reaching movements are defined with respect to terminal locations, then terminal locations could be used to *find* motor programs for reaching movements (e.g., if motor programs were organized in memory according to terminal locations), *supplied* to motor programs, or both. We may distinguish, therefore, between parameters for *finding* motor programs and parameters for *filling in* motor programs. An important goal of motor programming research is to identify which parameters are used in which programming process.

How can one attempt to achieve this goal? One approach is to seek evidence for prepackaged programs. Developmental research suggests that such programs exist, as innate movement patterns have been widely observed (e.g., Birnholz and Farrell 1984; Fentress 1973). Evidence for prepackaged programs is also abundant in the neurophysiological literature, where stimulation of single cells – so-called command neurons – has been found to produce stereotyped patterns of coordinated movement (DeLong 1971; Kupferman and Weiss 1978). Indirect evidence for such command neurons in man has also been offered by Rosenbaum (1977) and Heuer (1980), based on applications of the perceptual selective adaptation paradigm to motor performance.

Another way to learn about stored motor programs is to study transfer from one movement pattern to another. Summers (1975) trained subjects to press keys in response to sequences of lights presented in a fixed schedule. When subjects were later instructed to produce the key sequence from memory as quickly as possible but without regard to the time pattern they had originally learned, they could press the keys in the correct order and more quickly than before but not without a vestige of the original time pattern. Summers (1975) concluded that timing was represented as an integral part of the stored program for the key sequence.

Summers' conclusion relies on the preservation of invariant time relationships when subjects purposely change their speed of motor output. Terzuolo and Viviani (1980) discovered similar invariances in typing that were associated with small, spontaneous variations in typing speed. Based on constancies in the relative timing of successive keystrokes within highly practiced works, Terzuolo and Viviani argued that the production of such words is governed by prepackaged programs, an inference supported by an earlier training study by Leonard and Newman (1964). Timing invariances of this kind have also been used to argue for stored programs for writing (Viviani and Terzuolo 1980) and reaching (Jeannerod 1981).

Another approach to the analysis of program-finding and program-filling is to seek evidence for abstract programming variables. Such programming variables are presumably employed as arguments in motor programs, suggesting that one can learn about the basic structure of programs by identifying the arguments they take. Rumelhart and Norman (1982) argued for abstract program operators in the control of typewriting. Based on the fact that typists make mistakes such as typing *eroors* rather than *errors,* Rumelhart and Norman concluded that there is an abstract doubling operator which is applied (or misapplied) to keystroke commands. This conclusion agrees with the idea that abstract rules are used for rapid finger sequences (Collard and Povel 1982; Inhoff, Rosenbaum, Gordon, and Campbell 1984). Typing errors have also been used to infer the existence of abstract programming variables for individual keystrokes (Grudin 1983). The abstract programming variables of finger, hand, and finger trajectory were postulated on the basis of mirror-image errors in which individual keystrokes homologous to the ones intended were actually made (e.g., *e* instead of *i* on the *qwerty* keyboard).

Another source of evidence for abstract programming variables is the observation that neuronal discharge frequencies depend on specific, abstract properties of forthcoming movements. For example, Evarts (1967) found that discharge frequencies of motor cortex neurons in the monkey are related to the force and rate of change of force of forthcoming hand movements. Georgopolous et al. (1983) identified cells in the motor cortex whose discharge frequencies are related to the direction of imminent arm movements. Schiller and Koerner (1971), Sparks, Holland, and Guthrie (1976), and Wurtz and Goldberg (1972) found cells in the superior colliculus that fire differentially, depending on both the direction and the distance of forthcoming saccadic eye movements. The latter studies, showing effects of direction and distance, are particularly interesting because they appear to conflict with the conclusion, mentioned earlier in this chapter, that location is the key programming variable for saccades. Finding that motor programs are coded with respect to two redundant dimensions, such as target location on the one hand and direction and distance on the other, suggests that there are different stages in the movement programming process (see Arbib, Iberall, and Lyons 1983; Sparks and Mays 1983). Conceivably, direction and distance are used in finding motor programs while location is used in filling in motor programs that have already been found. Recently reported experiments that apply Rosenbaum's (1980) movement precuing technique to the analysis of saccade programming (Abrams and Jonides 1984) support this hypothesis.

A final source of evidence for abstract programming variables comes from reaction-time studies in which advance information about those variables is supplied to the subject before a reaction signal is presented (see Rosenbaum 1983 c, for review). The reasoning is that if subjects actually make use of a particular abstract programming variable, they should benefit from advance information about it. A broad range of studies has supported this basic hypothesis, although there has been controversy over methodological issues surrounding the use of this movement *precuing* technique (Goodman and Kelso 1980; Rosenbaum 1983 c). One general conclusion that these studies have supported, however, is that the defining characteristics of forthcoming movements need not be specified in a fixed order [see Rosenbaum (1983 c) for a review and Reeve and Proctor (1984) for a recent contribution]. A variable specification order may be used because this programming method allows for flexible *reprogramming* in movement correction and may allow for efficient programming of successive movements when only a few characteristics distinguish one movement from the next (Rosenbaum and Saltzman 1984).

Storage

If motor programs go through different stages, one might expect there to be corresponding memory stores as well. This issue constitutes another important question in the analysis of motor programming. Some investigators have argued for the existence of a special motor-command buffer (Henry and Rogers 1960; Morton 1970; Sternberg et al. 1978) while others have questioned its existence (Ehrlich and Cooper 1982; Rosenbaum, Inhoff, and Gordon 1984). No matter how this debate is resolved, there can be no doubt that limits exist on the size of motor programs that can be readied for execution. Although movements can be preprogrammed as far ahead as a second or more (Rosenbaum 1983 a; Shapiro 1977), the span of preprogramming is generally believed not to extend much beyond this point (Schmidt 1982). Likewise, in terms of the number of responses that can be preprogrammed, as opposed to the maximum duration over which preprogramming can extend, there is evidence for definite limits (Monsell and Nelson 1983).

Strictly speaking, it is not necessary to assume that the limits of preprogramming derive from limits on the capacity of program stores. Preprogramming limitations could also derive from lack of predictability about the success of forthcoming movements, in which case it might be inefficient to program too far into the future. Recent work by Rosenbaum et al. (1984) suggests, however, that there is a definite tendency to "save space" in motor programming. Subjects in these experiments chose between two possible finger sequences, with the relationship between the sequences varied across experimental conditions. When the two sequences shared responses up to a certain serial position the choice reaction time for the first response decreased with the position of the first uncertain response. If subjects simply prepared two separate programs for the two possible sequences, an effect of response context on choice reaction time would not have been expected. The tendency to combine programs from two possible sequences into one suggests that people try to minimize the storage requirements of programs that are about to be executed.

Learning

Following the discussion of how programs are stored just before execution, the question arises of how programs are learned and stored in long-term memory. As has already been suggested here, it is generally believed that motor programs stored in long-term memory are schematic (Bartlett 1932; Schmidt 1975) and are specified in increasing detail before being physically realized (cf., Keele 1981; Rosenbaum 1984). Because the focus of this chapter is on the cognitive substrates of movement genesis rather than on the acquisition of motor skills, I will eschew a detailed discussion of the extensive research that has been done on the learning of motor programs. Suffice it to say that this research has focused on the activities that allow for the formation and retention of the *motor schemas* or *generalized motor programs* that are believed to underlie skilled performance. The reader is referred to Schmidt (1982) for an extensive review of this literature.

Scheduling

As the review thusfar has indicated, many approaches have been taken in the study of motor programming, and a wide range of questions has been addressed. Clearly, a unifying framework is needed for work in this area. In the remainder of this chapter I suggest one possible framework. I do so by "returning to basics" and considering what sort of mechanism might allow for the serial ordering and timing of movements. I believe that the lack of a clear formulation of such a mechanism has hampered progress in this area.

The question of how movements are timed lies at the heart of the analysis of motor control. As Kelso (1981) has argued, timing is probably the most important parameter in all of movement control. The problem of timing is intimately related to the problem of serial order, the problem that occupied Lashley (1951) in his manifesto for motor programming research. When the delay between two responses has a particular arithmetic sign the order of the responses is also given. Thus, a mechanism that controls movement timing can also control serial order.

The main hypothesis I wish to offer is that a motor program is a *schedule* of motor events or, more precisely, a list of associations between labels for motor commands and clock pulses. Motor programming, according to this hypothesis, is the process of determining which motor commands are to be employed and with which clock pulses they are to be associated. Executing a motor program is the process of allowing responses to be triggered when their associated clock pulses occur. On this view, a motor program is like a printed schedule, say, of a train system. Such a schedule is an abstract representation of a desired course of actions. The times and locations listed in the schedule are abstract representations of actual times and places. Motor programs, by analogy, indicate which actions are to be performed when.

In the remainder of this chapter I review evidence that pertains to the scheduling view of motor programming. One virtue of the scheduling framework is that apparently disparate phenomena of motor performance can be understood as deriving from the same basic mechanism. In the final sections of the chapter I suggest an elaboration of the basic hypothesis that may provide a useful framework for future work in this area.

Evidence for Scheduling

What evidence can be adduced for the scheduling perspective? In this section I review evidence for the three core principles of the hypothesis, namely, that (1) there are abstract timing lists which guide movement production, (2) that associations are formed between response commands and identified clock pulses, and

(3) that the pulses of one or more running clocks pace the physical production of motor responses.

Abstract Timing Lists

The scheduling hypothesis maintains that abstract timing lists are used in movement production. One source of evidence for such abstract timing lists is the finding that timing is preserved despite changes in the conditions under which movements are performed. Conrad and Brooks (1974) trained monkeys to make rapid arm movements to and fro between two stops. When the distance between the stops was unexpectedly changed, the originally learned timing pattern of flexion and extension was preserved. Thus, the forces exerted by the extensors and flexors occurred at their original times despite the changed positions of the stops, suggesting that an autonomous schedule of extensor and flexor activity governed performance of the movement sequence. In fundamental agreement with this conclusion, Meyer et al. (1982) recently presented evidence for independent timing and force specifications for arm movements in humans.

Grudin (see Gentner and Norman 1984) identified errors in typing which suggest that there are separate representations for timing commands and muscle commands. He found that when transposition errors occurred in typing (e.g., *thme* rather than *them*) the normal timing of successive keystrokes is preserved (e.g., the *m* is typed when the *e* normally occurs and vice versa).

Additional support for abstract timing lists comes from choice reaction-time experiments. Klapp (1977b) found that subjects benefited from advance information about the duration of a forthcoming response (a Morse code "dit" or "dah") even if they did not know which muscles would be used to perform it (the thumb or index finger). This outcome is consistent with the assumption that the timing of movement sequences can be readied independently of the muscle commands needed to realize the timing. Klapp and Greim (1979) found that aimed hand movements requiring different durations for completion could not be prepared together. Similar results have been obtained by Heuer (1982a, b) and Rosenbaum et al. (1984). In the latter study it was found that uncertainty about the temporal structure of sequences to be produced had far more dramatic effects on choice reaction time than uncertainty about other characteristics of the sequences (e.g., which fingers to use). This result accords with the conclusion reached by Summers (1981) in his excellent review of motor programming, that "The specification of timing seems to play a special role in programming which is not shared by other components of a movement sequence, such as the spatial and muscular aspects" (pp. 57–58).

Associations Between Pulses and Response Commands

If, as the scheduling hypothesis assumes, associations are formed between clock pulse identifiers and response commands, then, to the extent that the associations strengthen with practice, it should be possible to observe invariant relations between the temporal and spatial characteristics of movement patterns. Such invariances have been observed. Armstrong (1970; see also Pew 1974) trained subjects to move a lever in the horizontal plane over a particular spatial and temporal course; visual feedback was provided to enable subjects to learn the desired spatiotemporal pattern. Armstrong found that after visual feedback was removed the phasing of movements was preserved despite spontaneous variations in the overall time to complete the task. Thus, the ratio of the time between the first leftward turn and the first rightward turn relative to the total time was approximately constant, the time between the first rightward turn and second leftward turn relative to the total time was approximately constant, and so on. A number of other investigators have obtained evidence for the same sort of phenomenon in lever movement tasks (Shapiro 1977), handwriting (Viviani and Terzuolo 1983), drawing (Lacquaniti, Terzuolo, and Viviani 1984), reaching (Jeannerod 1981), sequential button-pressing (Summers 1975), and typing (Terzuolo and Viviani 1979; but see Gentner 1982).

These demonstrations of space-time invariances suggest that strong associations are formed between clock pulse identifiers and instructions governing the spatial characteristics of movements. Informal demonstrations of such associations can also be found. Consider the act of singing. It is easy to replace the words of one song with the words of another. Try singing the melody of "Twinkle, twinkle, little star" but with the words of some other song, for example, "Mary had a little lamb." This task is easy, suggesting that lyrics and melody are dissociable. Now try to sing "Twinkle, twinkle, little star" retaining the rhythm but using the melody of "Mary had a little lamb." This task is almost impossible, regardless of whether words are included or not. Melody and rhythm therefore seem to be inextricably tied together in the production system, at least for songs that are highly practiced. In terms of the scheduling framework, this suggests that with practice strong associations are formed between the instructions that allow for melodic contour and those that allow for rhythm.

Another indirect source of evidence for associations between response commands and timing instructions comes from an area of research that has received relatively little attention from students of motor behavior – the study of verbal learning. A well-known theory emerging from this line of study originated with Ebbinghaus (1885/1964), the founder of verbal learning research. He theorized that memory traces of learned items are associated with one another in such a way that forward associations are stronger than backward associations and that the strength of association decreases with the distance of the items being associated. Problems with this theory were uncovered by Young (1959, 1968), who showed that when subjects learned a new list with a pair of items that should have been learned well according to Ebbinghaus' associative theory (e.g., WABZ after learning ABCD), the transfer from the old list to the new was not significantly better than in a control condition where none of the pairs in the new list had been previously studied (e.g., WABZ after WXYZ).

A possible replacement for Ebbinghaus' theory is that associations are formed between memory items and the serial positions they occupy. Several sources of evidence have been offered for this serial position hypothesis [see Crowder (1976) for review]. One is that subjects can report with a fair degree of accuracy where in a list of memory items specific items occur (Schulz 1955). Another is that intrusion errors from one list to another consist of items from corresponding serial positions more often than would be expected by chance (Fuchs and Melton 1974). Perhaps the most dramatic evidence comes from a study by Ebenholtz (1963). He first trained subjects on a list of the form ABCDEFGHIJ. Then his subjects learned one of three kinds of list: (1) *coordinate* lists, XBXDXFXHXJX; (2) *disparate* list, XHXJXBXDXFX; or (3) *control* lists, XXXXXXXXXXX, where X denotes fillers. Note that in the coordinate lists the preserved items occupy the same serial positions as in the original list, whereas in the disparate list this is not the case. Both lists retain their original forward associations and inter-item distances, however, suggesting that if serial position information plays no role in memory for serially ordered materials, transfer to the two types of list should be equal. In fact, performance in the coordinate condition was clearly superior to performance in the disparate condition. Moreover, performance in the disparate condition was no better than in the control conditon. Thus, contrary to Ebbinghaus' original "chaining" theory, Ebenholtz's data support a theory which allows that associations are formed between to-be-remembered items and their serial positions. This conclusion is consistent with the scheduling viewpoint offered here which posits associations between motor instructions and serial positions within a temporally structured series of production events. Of course, because the data just reviewed come from verbal recall tasks rather than "movement" tasks, they may not necessarily carry over to the movement system. On the other hand, the consistency of the conclusions from the two domains may reflect the accuracy of the scheduling hypothesis.

Clocks

According to the scheduling hypothesis, motor commands are triggered when their associated clock pulses occur. The idea that motor performance is based on the functioning of one or more central clocks has been advocated by Wing (1980), who proposed that motor timing is based on a central time-keeper that emits pulses periodically but with variability. In Wing's model, the delay between two reponses is controlled by the number of pulses between them. Because of the stochastic assumption in the model, as the delay increases so too should the variability of interresponse times. In fact this is what one observes. Figure 4 shows the result of a study by Rosenbaum and Patashnik (1980 b) in which subjects pressed a button with the left index finger followed by the right index finger to approximate a target delay. In a block of experimental trials the target delay was constant and was communicated to the subject through feedback that took the form of a vertical line presented at the end of each trial; the length of the line indicated how much the obtained delay deviated from the target delay, and the direction of the line indicated the direction of error. The variances of the pro-

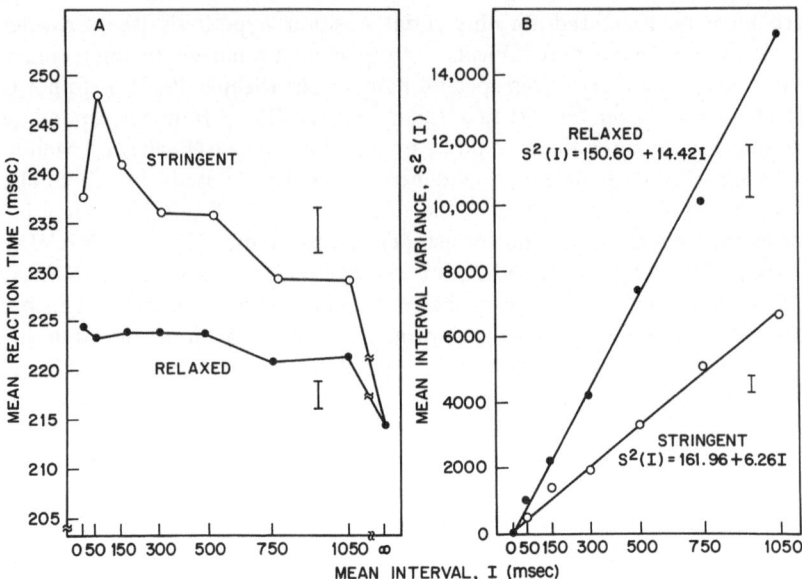

Fig. 4A, B. Mean latency of the first response (**A**) and mean variance of the interval between the first response and second (**B**) in the sequences studied by Rosenbaum and Patashnik (1980a). See text for details

duced delays increased with the means of the delays, as predicted by Wing's model.

In Wing's model, clock pulses serve two functions. One is to trigger responses; the other is to meter out delays between successive triggerings. Since particular pulses serve the trigger function, there must be some means of identifying or distinguishing them from nontrigger pulses. The data from the study of Rosenbaum and Patashnik bear on this point. As seen in the right-hand panel of Fig. 4, the slope of the variance function was larger in the "relaxed" condition than in the "stringent" condition. These conditions differed with respect to the degree of accuracy required, which was manipulated by changing the factor relating the length of the feedback line to the degree of interresponse time error. In the stringent condition, where small errors resulted in long lines, interresponse time variance increased with interresponse time mean at a slower rate than in the relaxed condition, where even large errors resulted in short lines.

A model that accounts for this result assumes that trigger pulses were more variable in the relaxed condition than in the stringent condition (see Rosenbaum and Patashnik 1980a; Rosenbaum 1983a). Suppose that before production of the two-response sequence, the identity of the trigger pulse for the second response was determined. With greater variability in the initially selected pulses, the produced intervals would also be more variable. If pulse identities were determined in advance, it is plausible to expect that the time taken to determine them would reflect the care of doing so. Thus, the time to determine pulse identities ahead of time should be inversely related to the variability of selected pulses. As it happens, the subjects in Rosenbaum and Patashnik's study were not only supposed to minimize the deviation of produced interresponse times from target interresponse times; they were also supposed to minimize the simple reaction time to make the first response after the appearance of an imperative signal. As seen in the left panel of Fig. 4, simple reaction time depended on the size of the interval to be produced and was longer in the stringent condition than in the relaxed condition. The reaction-time results can be accounted for with a quantitative model which assumes that "clock-setting" (i.e., determining the identity of the trigger pulse for the second response) took place before the first response sequence was performed. Specifically, as shown by Rosenbaum (1983a), simple reaction time was inversely related to the variance of number of clock pulses determined to occur between the first response and the second. That such a model accounts for the data suggests that the motor system is capable of labelling discrete clock pulses, as the scheduling hypothesis assumes.

Scheduling Hierarchies

Let us now consider how the scheduling framework helps account for the appearance of hierarchical control in the production of movement sequences. First, we will consider response timing. Then, we will consider errors.

Response Timing

Recall that earlier in this chapter I reviewed response timing evidence for the hierarchical control of rapid movement sequences based on response timing data from Rosenbaum et al. (1983) and Sternberg et al. (1978). A tree-traversal model was adducted to account for these results. At this point it is important to raise the question of how the tree-traversal process is assumed to be controlled. It is convenient to draw a tree and imagine control passing through it in a systematic fashion, but without a deeper explanatory principle for how the flow of control is itself governed more questions may be raised than answered. Crowder (1976), in discussing a tree-traversal model of serial recall proposed by Johnson (1970, 1972), made a similar observation: "the theory leaves many of the most fundamental problems – order tags, coding mechanisms, decoding mechanisms – shrouded in mystery" (p. 433). Crowder's criticism is just as telling for movement production as for serial recall.

How can Crowder's criticism be answered? Estes (1972) provided one plausible mechanism (see Fig. 5). In Estes' model, memory elements are organized hierarchically in such a way that superordinate elements make excitatory connections to subordinate elements and subordinate elements make unidirectional

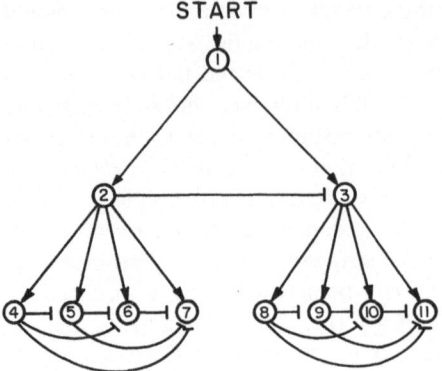

Fig. 5. Serial order mechanism that relies on excitatory connections (*arrows*) and inhibitory connections (*dashes*). (Based on Estes 1972)

inhibitory connections with one another. The larger the number of inhibitory connections impinging on a memory element the later it will be activated after excitation has been delivered from its corresponding superordinate element. Refractory delays (not shown in Fig. 5) affect elements that have been activated, making it possible for other elements to be produced. Thus, referring to Fig. 5, if element 1 delivers excitatory inputs to elements 2 and 3, element 2 will be activated first because it is less inhibited than element 3. Likewise, after element 2 excites elements 4, 5, 6, and 7, element 4 will be activated first and then become refractory, element 5 will be activated next and then become refractory, and so on. Once all the elements excited by element 2 have been activated, element 2 will itself become refractory and element 3 will take over.

Although Estes' model was introduced to account for data concerning serial recall, it is also applicable to the serial production of movements. Indeed, Rumelhart and Norman (1982) proposed a model for typing based on Estes' model.

Some difficulties with Estes' model arise, however, both in connection with its basic operation and in connection with its utility for response timing. First, it is unclear why when two elements receive excitatory inputs from the same superordinate element (e.g., elements 2 and 3 in Fig. 5) both elements do not fire immediately. Somehow, inhibition must build up on elements that are to fire later before the earlier elements fire.

Second, it is unclear how Estes' model accounts for the fact that the same memory elements can be produced in different orders when they occur in different well-learned sequences. One solution to this problem is to say that different tokens exist for the same memory elements and that different inhibitory connections exist among those tokens. However, this system requires as many tokens as serial orders for the same *n*-tuple of memory elements, a possibility that has been taken seriously by Wickelgren (1969) but that has been effectively dismissed by MacNeilage and Ladefoged (1976). Another more attractive possibility is that there is a system that dictates which inhibitory connections are to be made between the same memory elements, depending on the context in which those elements are to be produced.

A third difficulty with Estes' model is that it does not provide a clear method for controlling delays between correctly ordered serial elements. Such control is needed, for even when subjects try to "go as fast as possible" they in fact introduce controlled delays between responses (e.g., to avoid jamming keys on a mechanical typewriter). Moreover, one must consider what happens when people do not try to go as fast as possible but instead introduce prolonged delays between particular responses or modulate the overall rate of entire response sequences. The introduction of prolonged interresponse delays is of fundamental concern in the study of serial ordering, for when one considers what it means to say that a sequence has n responses (the principal independent variable in studies of sequence length effects), it is only by virtue of the length of the delay between the last response in the required sequence and the next response to be performed that the next response either "belongs" to the sequence or not.

Estes' mechanism would have to use varying amounts of inhibition between successive elements to ensure different delays between those elements. But it is unclear how, in different performance contexts, different delays could be placed between the same two responses – the same problem raised earlier in connection with serial order. Everyday experience shows that the timing of most response pairs does not become fixed with practice (e.g., a musician can freely vary the delay between two notes), although the phasing of extended sequences of responses may become firmly entrenched with practice (Summers 1975).

Following the lead of Summers' results, and following the impression of some investigators that, at least for skilled musicians, timing is specified independently of response identity (Shaffer 1982; J. A. Sloboda, personal communication, July 18, 1984), it is possible to consider a revised version of Estes' model that allows both for the extrinsic representation and flexible control of timing (see Fig. 6a). Unlike Estes' model, this *hierarchical delay* model incorporates clocks into the control hierarchy. Each clock, after its prescribed delay has transpired, can activate one or more clocks or one or more control elements, or the physical execution of muscle contractions or relaxations. Although it is not necessary to postulate feedback in such a system, adding it helps avoid timing errors resulting from random variation in the running of the clocks or errors in initial scheduling (i.e., errors in the delays specified for the clocks). Figure 6b shows how feedback can be used for this purpose. Here, each clock must receive input both from a superordinate control element and from the control element of the last performed response in order to begin. Note that the feedback imagined here does not necessarily rely on peripheral sensory pathways, although it is known that changes in peripheral feedback can affect timing performance (Wing 1977). Note also that if the processing of an input signal by a clock or control element is assumed to take at least one time unit, longer interresponse times should occur when more such elements must be traversed.

How can this form of representation be used to impose constraints on the movement sequences that can be performed? Figure 7 shows one possibility. This

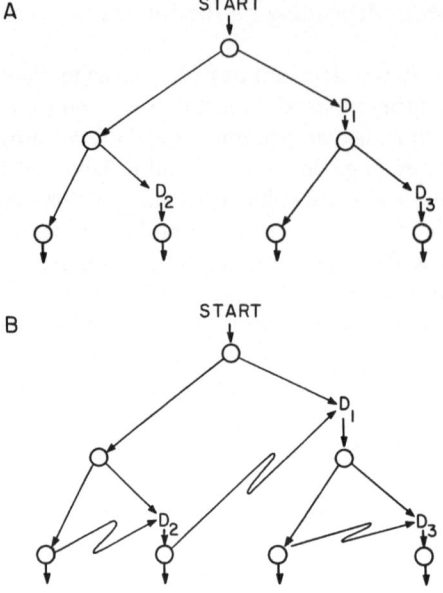

Fig. 6A, B. Hierarchical delay model without feedback (**A**) and with feedback (**B**). Excitation is issued in parallel to control elements (*circles*) and delayed elements (D_1, D_2, D_3)

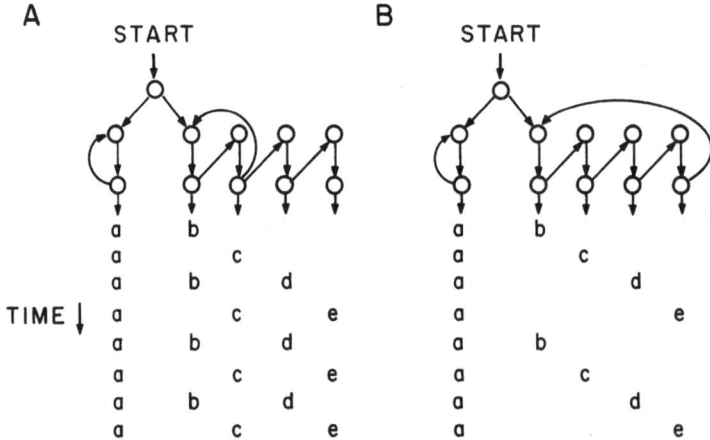

Fig. 7A, B. Delay line system for production of responses *a, b, c, d,* and *e* with the restart connection for *bcde* emanating from *c* in **A** and from *e* in **B**. Here each column consists of two units, but one unit or more than two units could make up each column, in which case the period of the system would be changed correspondingly

is a delay-line system (cf. Kornhuber 1975) where miniature delay elements (e.g., neurons) are strung together in an orderly fashion. Assuming that there is a fixed delay between the receipt and release of a signal by any such element, delays of varying length can be produced by introducing varying numbers of elements into the delay line. For example, by placing the connection that restarts the right-hand part of the network at different points in the network (or equivalently, by potentiating a desired preexisting connection), it is possible to vary the delay between the restart of the *bcde* subsequence without affecting the times between *b* and *c, c* and *d,* and *d* and *e* (see Fig. 7). Note that the cycle time of the right-hand part of the network is always an integral multiple of the cycle time of the left-hand part of the network and therefore is a "higher-level" clock.

More work with networks of this kind is needed to determine why some timing relationships are harder than others. It is quite easy to vary the delay between successive renditions of a fixed movement sequence, perhaps because, as suggested in Fig. 7, all that is needed is a change in the position of the restart connection. It is much harder, as any musician can attest and Cohen (1970), Klapp (1979), and Peters (1977) have shown formally, to produce harmonically unrelated movements simultaneously. Likewise, people apparently find it difficult to perform bimanual aiming movements with asynchronous starts and finishes (Kelso, Southard, and Goodman 1979). Constraints in delay line networks and/or their connections to control elements will have to be found to account for limitations of this kind. One avenue for discovering such constraints may be the statistical analysis of response timing, using the elegant analytic tools developed by Vorberg and Hambuch (1978) for distinguishing between hierarchical and linear timing networks.

Errors

The scheduling framework suggested here also provides a way of accounting for errors in motor performance. Recall that the hypothesis says there are two main stages of motor programming: (1) determining which motor instructions should be used and with which clock pulses they should be associated and (2) allowing the motor instructions to be triggered when their corresponding clock pulses occur. Each of these stages introduces opportunities for different types of error. Stage 1 allows for incorrect selections of motor instructions and clock pulses. Stage 2 allows for errors of execution.

To see how the scheduling framework accounts for the sorts of errors that have been observed in actual production, consider the spoonerism – the error of reversing syllable-initial phonemes of neighboring stressed syllables. A well-known example is "You hissed all my mystery lectures" instead of "You missed all my history lectures." This error is explained as follows in the scheduling framework. Suppose that the scheduled times for the /m/ in *missed* and the /h/ in *history* share the same low-level clock identifiers. For instance, suppose that /m/ is scheduled to occur at time 1:03 and /h/ is scheduled to occur at time 2:03, where the numbers to the left of the colon denote high-level clock values and the numbers to the right denote low-level clock values. Suppose that in preparing for stage 2 an error is made of reversing the high-level clock identifiers for /m/ and /h/; /m/ is assigned 2:03 and /h/ is assigned 1:03. The result is the exchange of /m/ and /h/.

This example illustrates how speech errors can be accounted for in the scheduling framework. It remains for later research to show how the framework can account in more detail for a wider range of slips of the tongue and why only particular sorts of errors occur. Nonetheless, it is worth mentioning that an appealing feature of the scheduling position is that it provides a clear mechanism for producing exchanges and other sorts of speech errors. In the past, with few exceptions (Dell and Reich 1980), accounts of speech errors have been vague about why different elements exchange, blend, and so on, primarily because the investigators concerned with such errors have been more interested in the linguistic structures suggested by them than in the processes that produce them (cf. Fromkin 1980).

Scheduling also provides a basis for error analysis outside the speech realm. Take the rapid key-pressing study by Rosenbaum et al. (1983). The error data, like the timing data, could be accounted for with a tree-traversal model. The explanatory principle for the error data was that control passed down the wrong branch of the tree. The scheduling framework provides an alternative way of conceptualizing such errors. The mechanism is the assignment of clock pulses to motor instructions. Incorrect clock pulse assignments would cause responses to occur at the wrong time, and the greater the similarity between clock pulse identifiers for two responses, the higher the likelihood of confusion between them. Grudin's data concerning transposition errors in typing fit perfectly with this idea. Recall that when he found reversals in the serial positions of keystrokes within words (e.g., *thme* rather than *them*) the timing profile of the word was essentially unchanged from its normal form. In future developments of the scheduling framework, it will be important to pay close attention to performance errors to test and motivate particular assumptions of the models being considered.

Concluding Remarks

Let us review the main points of this chapter. First, I defended the intentional framework for analyzing motor performance, arguing that the diversity of performance produced in the same stimulus conditions requires the ascription of flexible programming abilities to the actor. Next, I reviewed the definitions that have been given for the term motor program and the evidence that has been adduced for motor programming. I turned then to the principal questions that have been addressed in motor programming research, all of which bear directly or indirectly on the structure of motor programs and the characteristics of the information-processing system that allows for their storage, retrieval, construction, and execution. In the final sections of the chapter, I offered a scheduling framework for modelling motor programs which takes as its starting point the central importance of timing in movement control. Building on the idea that timing can be abstractly represented in advance of movement execution, the main hypothesis offered was that a motor program is a hierarchical list of associations between commands and clock pulses. The list is hierarchical in the sense that commands and clock pulses can control other commands and clock pulses as well as the associations between them. It was shown that a hierarchical scheduling system can account for results concerning serial recall, space-time invariance, reaction time, timing variability, and errors in sequential performance. In discussing how schedules might be implemented neuronally, it was shown that delay-line systems could provide waits of various lengths as well as patterns of timing relationships among simultaneously and successively produced movements. Considerable work is still needed in this area, however, to provide a more rigorous account of the timing mechanisms that both allow for and limit various sorts of motor performance.

In closing, I would like to offer some general comments on the current state of research in the area of motor programming. As the present review has indicated, the approaches that have been taken to this topic are multifaceted. So too are the theoretical orientations and commitments of workers in this area. As with all such differences in an important area of study, the arguments will no doubt foster a deeper understanding. But for this to happen it will become increasingly important for the parties involved to listen to each other with a constructive as well as a critical attitude. I believe, too, that the scope of our inquiry will have to broaden to benefit from, and in turn shed light on, some domains of research that so far have been largely ignored.

One of these areas is robotics, where the need for practical solutions to problems of programming and coordination has given rise to explicit formulations of adaptive control. As various strategies for robot movement are developed (cf., Hinton, 1984), it will be important to see how well they apply to biological control. Likewise, the principles employed by animals (including man) should inform the design of artificial control systems.

Another area that should be heeded more carefully by motor psychologists is linguistics, where the search for rules limiting allowable output has become increasingly successful over recent years. Developing a "grammar of action" is likely to be an important goal of future work. The principal challenge here will be to infer the rules used in selecting voluntary movements.

Finally, the clinical domain is another that must be attended to more by students of motor programming. Disorders of movement, especially disorders involving high-level functions, are likely to provide important clues into the normal control of movement, as several groups of investigators have already noted (e.g., Margolin and Wing 1983). Perhaps of greater importance is that as our basic understanding of movement control grows, so too should our ability to help those for whom normal movement is difficult.

Acknowledgments. Parts of this chapter were written while the author was on a sabbatical visit to the MIT Center for Cognitive Science. Preparation of the chapter was supported in part by grants BNS-8120104 and BNS-8408634 from the National Science Foundation, by Research Career Development Award 1 KO4 NS00942-01 from the National Instituts of Health and by the MIT Center for Cognitive Science under a grant from the A. P. Sloan Foundation's Particular Program in Cognitive Science. The author thanks Craig Bonner, George Cobb, William Estes, Herbert Heuer, Neil Stillings, and an anonymous reviewer for helpful comments.

References

Abrams, R. J., and Jonides, J. (1984). Programming saccadic eye movements. Paper presented at the 25th Annual Meeting of Psychonomic Society, San Antonio, Texas.

Adams, J. A. (1976). Issues for a closed-loop theory of motor learning. In G. E. Stelmach (Ed.), Motor control: Issues and trends (pp. 87–107). New York: Academic.

Arbib, M. A., Iberall, T., and Lyons, D. (1985). Coordinated control programs for movements of the hand. COINS Technical Report 83-25. University of Massachusetts, Amherst, Massachusetts. In A. W. Goodwin, I. Darian-Smith (Eds.), Hand function and the neocortex. New York: Springer (Experimental brain research supplement, Vol. 10) (in press).

Armstrong, T. R. (1970). *Training for the production of memorized movement patterns.* (Technical Report No. 26). Ann Arbor: University of Michigan, Human Performance Center.

Bartlett, F. C. (1932). *Remembering.* London: Cambridge University Press.

Birnholz, J. C., and Farrell, E. E. (1984). Ultrasound images of human fetal development. *American Scientist, 72,* 608–613.

Cohen, L. (1970). Interaction between limbs during bimanual voluntary activity. *Brain, 93,* 259–272.

Collard, R., and Povel, D.-J. (1982). Theory of serial pattern production: tree traversals. *Psychological Review, 85,* 693–707.

Conrad, B., and Brooks, V. B. (1974). Effects of dentate cooling on rapid alternating arm movements. *Journal of Neurophysiology, 37,* 792–804.

Crowder, R. G. (1976). *Principles of learning and memory.* Hillsdale, N. J.: Erlbaum.

Deecke, L., Grözinger, B., and Kornhuber, H. H. (1976). Voluntary finger movements in man: Cerebral potentials and theory. *Biological Cybernetics, 23,* 99–119.

Dell, G. S., and Reich, P. A. (1980). Toward a unified model of slips of the tongue. In V. A. Fromkin (Ed.), *Errors in linguistic performance* (pp. 273–286). New York: Academic.

DeLong, M. R. (1971). Central patterning of movement. *Neuroscience Research Program Bulletin, 9,* 10–30.

Ebbinghaus, H. E. (1885/1964). *Memory: A contribution to experimental psychology.* New York: Dover (Originally published 1885, translated 1913).

Ebenholtz, S. M. (1963). Position mediated transfer between serial learning and a spatial discrimination task. *Journal of Experimental Psychology, 65,* 603–608.

Ehrlich, S. F., and Cooper, W. E. (1982). Memory determinants of response latency to produce speech. *Acta Psychologica, 50,* 127–142.

Estes, W. K. (1972). An associative basis for coding and organization in memory. In A. W. Melton and E. Martin (Eds.), *Coding processes in human memory* (pp. 161–190). Washington, D. C.: Winston.

Evarts, E. V. (1967). Representation of movement and muscles by pyramidal tract neurons of the precentral motor cortex. In M. D. Yahr and D. P. Purpura (Eds.), *Neurophysiological basis of normal and abnormal motor activities.* New York: Raven.

Evarts, E. V. (1984). Neurophysiological approaches to brain mechanisms for preparatory set. In S. Kornblum and J. Requin (Eds.), *Preparatory states and processes.* Hillsdale, NJ: Erlbaum.

Evarts, E. V., Bizzi, E., Burke, R. E., DeLong, M., and Thach, W. T., Jr. (1971). Central control of movement. *Neurosciences Research Program Bulletin,* Vol. 9, No. 1.

Fel'dman, A. G. (1966). Functional tuning of the nervous system with control of movement or maintenance of a steady posture: II. Controllable parameters of the muscles. *Biophysics, 11,* 565–578.

Fentress, J. C. (1973). Development of grooming in mice with amputated forelimbs. *Science, 179,* 704–705.

Forssberg, H., Grillner, S., and Rossignol, S. (1975). Phasic gain control of reflexes from the dorsum of the paw during spinal locomotion. *Brain Research, 132,* 121–139.

Fromkin, V. A. (Ed.) (1980). *Errors in linguistic performance.* New York: Academic.

Fuchs, A. F. and Melton, A. W. (1974). Effects of frequency of presentation and stimulus length on retention in the Brown-Peterson paradigm. *Journal of Experimental Psychology, 103,* 629–637.

Gentner, D. R. (1982). Evidence against a central control model of timing in typing. *Journal of Experimental Psychology: Human Perception and Performance, 8,* 793–810.

Gentner, D. R. and Norman, D. A. (1984). The typist's touch. *Psychology Today, 3,* 66–72.

Georgopoulos, A. P., Caminiti, R., Kalaska, J. F., and Massey, J. T. (1983). Spatial coding of movement: A hypothesis concerning the coding of movement direction by motor cortical populations. In J. Massion, J. Paillard, W. Schultz, and M. Wiesendanger (Eds.), *Neural coding of motor performance.* New York: Springer-Verlag. (Experimental brain research supplementum, vol 7).

Goodman, D. and Kelso, J. A. S. (1980). Are movements prepared in parts? Not under compatible (naturalized) conditions. *Journal of Experimental Psychology: General, 109,* 475–495.

Grudin, J. G. (1983). Error patterns in novice and skilled typists. In W. E. Cooper (Ed.), *Cognitive aspects of skilled typewriting* (pp. 121–143). New York: Springer.

Guthrie, B. L., Porter, J. D., and Sparks, D. L. (1983). Corollary discharge provides accurate eye position to the oculomotor position. *Science 221,* 1193–1195.

Henry, F. M. and Rogers, D. E. (1960). Increased response latency for complicated movements and a "memory drum" theory of neuromotor reaction. *Research Quarterly, 31,* 448–458.

Heuer, H. (1980). Selective fatigue in the human motor system. *Psychological Research, 41,* 345–354.

Heuer, H. (1982a). Binary choice reaction time as a criterion of motor equivalence. *Acta Psychologica, 50,* 35–47.

Heuer, H. (1982b). Binary choice reaction time as a criterion of motor equivalence: Further evidence. *Acta Psychologica, 50,* 49–60.

Hinton, G. (1984). Parallel computations for controlling an arm. *Journal of Motor Behavior, 16,* 171–194.

Inhoff, A. W., Rosenbaum, D. A., Gordon, A. W., and Campbell, J. A. (1984). Stimulus–response compatibility and motor programming of manual response sequences. *Journal of Experimental Psychology: Human Perception and Performance, 10,* 724–733.

Jeannerod, M. (1981). Intersegmental coordination during reaching at natural objects. In J. Long and A. Baddeley (Eds.), *Attention and performance IX (pp. 153–169). Hillsdale, N.J.: Erlbaum.*

Jeannerod, M. (1984). How do we direct our actions in space? In A. Hein and M. Jeannerod (Eds.), *Spatially oriented behavior.* New York: Springer.

Johnson, N. F. (1970). The role of chunking and organization in the process of recall. In G. H. Bower (Ed.), *Psychology of learning and motivation, Vol. 4.* New York: Academic.

Johnson, N. F. (1972). Organization and the concept of a memory code. In A. W. Melton and E. Martin (Eds.), *Coding processes in human memory* (pp. 125–159). Washington, D.C.: Winston.

Keele, S. W. Movement control in skilled motor performance. *Psychological Bulletin, 70,* 387–403.

Keele, S. W. Behavioral analysis of movement control. In V. Brooks (Ed.), *Handbook of physiology: Motor control.* Washington, D. C.: American Physiological Society.

Kelso, J. A. S. (1981). Contrasting perspectives on order and regulation in movement. In J. Long and A. Baddeley (Eds.), *Attention and performance IX.* Hillsdale, NJ: Erlbaum.

Kelso, J. A. S. (Ed.) (1982). *Human motor behavior: An introduction.* Hillsdale, NJ: Erlbaum.

Kelso, J. A. S., Southard, D. L., and Goodman, D. (1979). On the co-ordination of two-handed movements. *Journal of Experimental Psychology: Human Perception and Performance, 5,* 229–238.

Kelso, J. A. S., Tuller, B., and Harris, K. S. (1983). A "dynamic pattern" perspective on the control and coordination of movement. In P. F. MacNeilage (Ed.), *The production of speech.* New York: Springer

Kent, R. D., and Minifie, F. D. (1977). Coarticulation in recent speech production models. *Journal of Phonetics, 5,* 115–133.

Kerr, B. A. (1978). Task factors that influence selection and preparation for voluntary movements. In G. E. Stelmach (Ed.), *Information processing in motor control and learning* (pp. 55–69). New York: Academic.

Klapp, S. T. (1977a). Reaction time analysis of programmed control. *Exercise and sport sciences reviews, 5,* 231–253.

Klapp, S. T. (1977b). Response programming, as assessed by reaction time, does not establish commands for particular muscles. *Journal of Motor Behavior, 9,* 301–312.

Klapp, S. T. (1979). Doing two things at once: The role of temporal compatibility. *Memory and Cognition, 7,* 375–381.

Klapp, S. T., and Greim, D. M. (1979). Programmed control of aimed movements revisited: The role of target visibility and symmetry. *Journal of Experimental Psychology: Human Perception and Performance, 5,* 509–521.

Klein, R. (1983). Nonhierarchical control of rapid movement sequences: A comment on Rosenbaum, Kenny, and Derr. *Journal of Experimental Psychology: Human Perception and Performance, 9,* 834–836.

Kornhuber, H. H. (1975). Cerebral cortex, cerebellum, and basal ganglia: an introduction to their motor functions. In E. V. Evarts (Ed.) *Central processing of sensory input leading to motor output.* Cambridge, MA: MIT Press

Kupferman, I., and Weiss, K. R. (1978). The command neuron concept. *The Behavioral and Brain Sciences, 1,* 3–39.

Lacquanti, F., Terzuolo, C., Viviani, P. (1984). Global metric properties and preparatory processes in drawing movements. In S. Kornblum and J. Requin (Eds.) *Preparatory states and processes* (pp. 357–370). Hillsdale, NJ: Erlbaum.

Lashley, K. S. (1917). The accuracy of movement in the absence of excitation from the moving organ. *American Journal of Physiology, 43,* 169–194.

Lashley, K. S. (1951). The problem of serial order in behavior. In L. A. Jeffress (Ed.), *Cerebral mechanisms in behavior* (pp. 112–131). New York: Wiley.

Leonard, J. A., & Newman, R. C. (1964). Formation of higher habits. *Nature, 203,* 550–551.

MacNeilage, P. F. (1970). Motor control of serial ordering of speech. *Psychological Review, 77,* 182–196.

MacNeilage, P. F. and Ladefoged, P. (1976). The production of speech and language. In C. Carterette & M. P. Friedman (Eds.), *Handbook of perception* (pp. 75–120). New York: Academic.

Margolin, D. I., and Wing, A. M. (1983). Agraphia and micrographia: Clinical manifestations of motor programming and performance disorders. *Acta Psychologica, 54,* 263–283.

Marteniuk, R. G., and MacKenzie, C. L. (1980). Information processing in movement organization and execution. In R. S. Nickerson (Ed.), *Attention and performance VIII* (pp. 29–57). Hillsdale, NJ: Erlbaum.

Merton, P. A. (1972). How we control the contraction of our muscles. *Scientific American, 226,* 5, 30–37.

Meyer, D. E., Smith, J. E. K., and Wright, C. E. (1982). Models for the speed and accuracy of aimed movements. *Psychological Review, 89,* 449–482.

Miller, G. A., Galanter, E., and Pribram, H. H. (1960). *Plans and the structure of behavior.* New York: Holt, Rinehart, and Winston.

Miller, J. (1982). Discrete versus continuous stage models of human information processing. *Journal of Experimental Psychology: Human Perception and Performance, 8,* 273–296.

Monsell, S., and Nelson, E. (1983). *Control of rapid speech: Limits on utterance programming capacity.* Paper presented at the twenty-fourth annual meeting of the Psychonomic Society, San Diego, CA.

Morton, J. (1970). A functional model for memory. In D. A. Norman (Ed.), *Models of human memory* (pp. 203–254). New York: Academic.

Peters, M. (1977). Simultaneous performance of two activities: The factor of timing. *Neuropsychologia, 15,* 461–465.

Pew, R. W. (1974). Human perceptual–motor performance. In B. H. Kantowitz (Ed.), *Human information processing: Tutorials in performance and cognition* (pp. 1–39). Hillsdale, NJ: Erlbaum.

Pew, R. W. (1984). A distributed processing view of human motor control. In W. Prinz and A. F. Sanders (Eds.) *Cognition and motor processes* (pp. 19–27). Berlin: Springer.

Polit, A. and Bizzi, E. (1978). Processes controlling arm movements in monkeys. *Science, 201,* 1235–1237.

Povel, D.-J., and Collard, R. (1982). Structural factors in patterned finger tapping. *Acta Psychologica, 52,* 107–124.

Powers, W. T. (1973). *Behavior: The control of perception.* Chicago: Aldine.

Reeve, T. G., and Proctor, R. W. (1984). On the advance preparation of discrete finger responses. *Journal of Experimental Psychology: Human Perception and Performance, 10,* 541–553.

Reitman, J. S. (1974). Without surreptitious rehearsal, information in short-term memory decays. *Journal of Verbal Learning and Verbal Behavior, 13,* 365–377.

Requin, J., Lecas, J-C., and Bonnet, M. (1984). Some experimental evidence for a three-step model of motor preparation. In S. Kornblum and J. Requin (Eds.), *Preparatory states and processes.* Hillsdale, NJ: Erlbaum.

Rosenbaum, D. A. (1977). Selective adaptation of "command neurons" in the human motor system. *Neuropsychologia, 15,* 81–91.

Rosenbaum, D. A. (1980). Human movement initiation: Specification of arm, direction, and extent. *Journal of Experimental Psychology: General, 109,* 444–474.

Rosenbaum, D. A. (1983a). Central control of movement timing. *The Bell System Technical Journal (Special Human Factors and Behavioral Sciences issue), 62,* 1647–1657.

Rosenbaum, D. A. (1983b). Hierarchical versus nonhierarchical models of movement sequence control: A reply to Klein. *Journal of Experimental Psychology: Human Perception and Performance, 9,* 837–839.

Rosenbaum, D. A. (1983c). The movement precuing technique: Assumptions, applications, and extensions. In R. A. Magill (Ed.) *Memory and control of action* (pp. 231–274). Amsterdam: North-Holland.

Rosenbaum, D. A. (1984). Planning and control of movement. In J. R. Anderson and S. M. Kosslyn (Eds.) *Tutorials in learning and memory: Essays in honor of Gordon Bower* (pp. 219–233). San Francisco: W. H. Freeman.

Rosenbaum, D. A., Kenny, S., and Derr, M. A. (1983). Hierarchical control of rapid movement sequences. *Journal of Experimental Psychology: Human Perception and Performance, 9,* 86–102.

Rosenbaum, D. A., Inhoff, A. W., and Gordon, A. M. (1984). Choosing between movement sequences: A hierarchical editor model. *Journal of Experimental Psychology: General, 113,* 372–393.

Rosenbaum, D. A. and Patashnik, O. (1980a). A mental clock-setting process revealed by reaction times. In G. E. Stelmach and J. Requin (Eds.), *Tutorials in motor behavior.* Amsterdam: North-Holland.

Rosenbaum, D. A. and Patashnik, O. (1980b). Time to time in the human motor system. In R. S. Nickerson (Ed.), *Attention and performance VIII* (pp. 93–106). Hillsdale, NJ: Erlbaum.

Rosenbaum, D. A. and Saltzman, E. (1984). A motor-program editor. In W. Prinz and A. Sanders (Eds.) *Cognition and motor processes* (pp. 51–61). Berlin: Springer.

Rumelhart, D. E. and Norman, D. A. (1982). Simulating a skilled typist: A study of skilled cognitive–motor performance. *Cognitive Science, 6,* 1–36.

Salthouse, T. A. (1984). The skill of typing. *Scientific American, 250,* 2, 128–135.

Schiller, P. H. and Koerner, F. (1971). Discharge characteristics of single units in superior colliculus of the alert rhesus monkey. *Journal of Neurophysiology, 34,* 920–936.

Schmidt, R. A. (1975). A schema theory of discrete motor skill learning. *Psychological Review, 82,* 225–260.

Schmidt, R. A. (1982). *Motor control and learning.* Champaign, IL: Human Kinetics.

Schneider, W. and Fisk, A. D. (1983). Attention theory and mechanisms for skilled performance. In R. A. Magill (Ed.) *Memory and control of action* (pp. 119–143). Amsterdam: North-Holland.

Schulz, R. W. (1955). Generalization of serial position in role serial learning. *Journal of Experimental Psychology, 49,* 267–272.

Shaffer, L. H. (1976). Intention and performance. *Psychological Review, 83,* 375–493.

Shaffer, L. H. (1982). Rhythm and timing in skill. *Psychological Review, 89,* 109–122.

Shapiro, D. C. (1977). A preliminary attempt to determine the duration of a motor program. In D. M. Landers and R. W. Christina (Eds.), *Psychology of motor behavior and sport* (Vol. 1). Champaign, IL: Human Kinetics.

Sparks, D. L. and Mays, L. E. (1983). Role of the monkey superior colliculus in the spatial localization of saccade targets. In A. Hein and M. Jeannerod (Eds.), *Spatially oriented behavior.* New York: Springer.

Sparks, D. L., Holland, R., and Guthrie, B. L. (1976). Size and distribution of movement fields in the monkey superior colliculus. *Brain Research, 113,* 21–34.

Sternberg, S., Monsell, S., Knoll, R. L., and Wright, C. E. (1978). The latency and duration of rapid movement sequences: Comparisons of speech and typewriting. In G. E. Stelmach (Ed.) *Information processing in motor control and learning* (pp. 117–152). New York: Academic.

Summers, J. J. (1975). The role of timing in motor program representation. *Journal of Motor Behavior, 7,* 229–241.

Summers, J. J. (1981). Motor programming. In D. H. Holding (Ed.), *Motor skills* (pp. 42–64). Chichester: Wiley.

Taub, E., and Berman, A. J. (1968). Movement and learning in the absence of sensory feedback. In S. J. Freeman (Ed.), *The neuropsychology of spatially oriented behavior* (pp. 173–192). Homewood, IL: Dorsey.

Terzuolo, C. A., and Viviani, P. (1979). The central representation of learning motor programs. In R. E. Talbot and D. R. Humphrey (Eds.), *Posture and movement. New York:* Raven.

Terzuolo, C. A., and Viviani, P. (1980). Determinants and characteristics of motor patterns used for typing. *Neuroscience, 5,* 1085–1103.

Teulings, H.-L., Thomassen, A. J., and van Galen, G. P. (1983). Preparation of partly pre-cued handwriting movements: The size of movement units in handwriting. *Acta Psychologica, 54,* 165–177.

Turvey, M. T. (1977). Preliminaries to a theory of action with reference to vision. In R. Shaw and J. Bransford (Eds.), *Perceiving, acting, and comprehending: Towards an ecological psychology.* Hillsdale, NJ: Erlbaum.

Van Galen, G. P., and Teulings, H.-L. (1983). The independent monitoring of form and scale factors in handwriting. *Acta Psychologica, 54,* 9–22.

Viviani, P., and Terzuolo, C. A. (1980). Space–time invariance in learned motor skills. In G. E. Stalmach and J. Requin (Eds.) *Tutorials in motor behavior* (pp. 525–533). Amsterdam: North-Holland.

Viviani, P., and Terzuolo, V. (1983). The organization of movement in handwriting and typing. In B. Butterworth (Ed.) *Language production* (Vol. 2). New York: Academic.

Volkmann, F. C., Schick, A. M., and Riggs, L. A. (1969). Time course of visual inhibiton during voluntary saccades. *Journal of the Optical Society of America, 58,* 562–569.

Volkmann, F. C., Riggs, L. A., and Moore, R. K. (1980). Eyeblinks and visual suppression. *Science, 207,* 900–902.

Vorberg, D. and Hambuch, R. (1978). On the temporal control of rhythmic performance. In J. Requin (Ed.) *Attention and performance VII* (pp. 533–555). Hillsdale, NJ: Erlbaum.

Wickelgren, W. A. (1969). Context-sensitive conding, associative memory, and serial order in (speech) behavior. *Psychological Review, 76,* 1–15.

Wing, A. (1977). Perturbation of auditory feedback delay and the timing of movement. *Journal of Experimental Psychology: Human Perception and Performance, 3,* 175–186.

Wing, A. (1980). The long and short of timing in response sequences. In G. E. Stelmach and J. Requin (Eds.) *Tutorials in motor behavior.* Amsterdam: North-Holland.

Wurtz, R. H. and Goldberg, M. E. (1972). Activity of the superior colliculus in behaving monkey. III. Cells discharging before eye movements. *Journal of Neurophysiology, 35,* 575–586.

Young, R. K. (1959). A comparison of two methods of learning serial associations. *American Journal of Psychology, 72,* 554–559.

Young, R. K. (1968). Serial learning. In T. R. Dixon and D. L. Horton (Eds.), *Verbal behavior and general behavior theory* (pp. 122–148). Englewood Cliffs, NJ: Prentice-Hall.

Waiting to Respond:
Electrophysiological Measurements in Man During Preparation for a Voluntary Movement

C. H. M. Brunia, S. A. V. M. Haagh, and J. G. M. Scheirs

Contents

Introduction

Waiting for the moment to react to an impending stimulus is accompanied by electrophysiological processes in the central nervous system (CNS) that can be measured from the surface of the body. In this chapter we will discuss electroencephalographic (EEG) and electromyographic (EMG) changes related to preparation for a movement. Most of the results originate from fixed foreperiod reaction time (RT) experiments. When a subject is informed about the moment the imperative (reaction) stimulus (RS) will be presented, the RT is shorter than when the subject is not informed. This information is provided by a warning stimulus (WS), with which the foreperiod starts. The WS has to be detected by the subject. Its significance has to be evaluated and a decision has to be made to prepare for the response. This preparation for the response might imply the presence of processes such as time estimation, anticipation, and response programming. The information processing in the CNS which takes place during the foreperiod and which results in the final response is reflected in electrophysiological changes at two different levels of the CNS: the cortex and the spinal cord. Although all kinds of subcortical and brain stem structures play an important role in the preparation for and the execution of movements, the cortical and spinal electrophysiological changes are the only ones which can be recorded from the surface of the body.

We will start our description of the electrophysiological changes with EEG data reflecting processes at the cortical level. Later on we will discuss some recent studies of changes in the excitability of motoneurons in the spinal cord. Finally we will try to understand how cortical and spinal changes might be interrelated.

The Cortical Level

Contingent Negative Variation

In 1964 Walter, Cooper, Aldridge, McCallum, and Winter reported a slow negative wave in the EEG during a 1-s foreperiod of a simple RT experiment. Repeated presentation of a stimulus results in an evoked response, which can be made visible with a proper averaging technique. If a pair of stimuli with an interval of 1 s are repeatedly presented, two evoked responses are visible, as can be seen in Figure 1. If the subject receives the instruction to react as quickly as possible after the second stimulus, a slow negative wave emerges from the background EEG during the interstimulus interval. This slow wave has been called contingent negative variation (CNV). Initially, it was related to the fact that the subject was expecting the RS. Hence the term expectancy (E) wave was coined. From the beginning of this line of research it has been a matter of debate whether a motor response to RS is crucial for the CNV to appear. Apart from the motor aspects, the CNV has been related to a number of different psychological or physiological processes. Among these were stress (Knott and Irwin 1973), motivation (Irwin, Knott, McAdam and Rebert 1966; Borda 1970), level of emotionality (Knott and Irwin 1973), attention (Hillyard and Galambos 1967; McCallum and Walter 1968), conation (Low, Borda, Frost and Kellaway 1966), and arousal (Tecce 1972).

When bilateral EEG recordings were made a symmetrical distribution of the CNV over both hemispheres was generally found. In the anterior-posterior axis the largest amplitudes were recorded at the vertex, smaller amplitudes in the frontal areas, and the smallest in the posterior region (Walter 1967; Cohen 1969). However, Low et al. (1966) reported larger amplitudes over the frontal sites. Such contrasting results, possibly related to different experimental designs, suggested that the CNV is not a unitary phenomenon, generated by one single brain mechanism. It might, on the contrary, represent a family of task-specific potentials, each indicating a different function and, therefore, possibly being related to different brain mechanisms (Hillyard 1973). An indication of this can be found in a paper by Järvilehto and Frühstorfer (1970), who distinguished be-

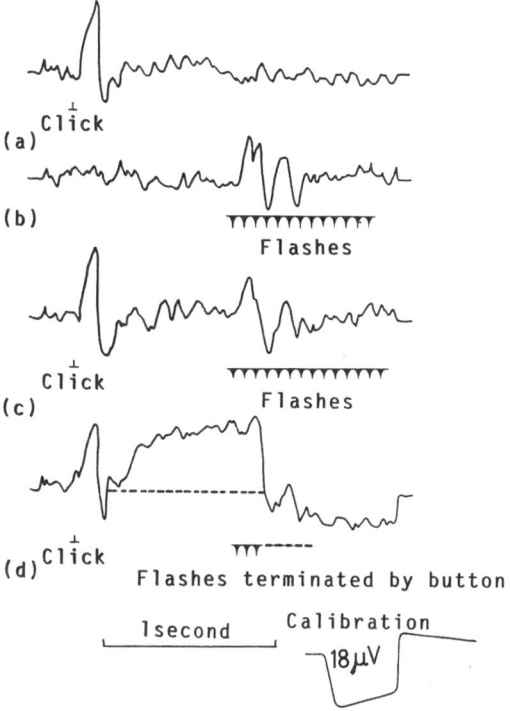

Fig. 1. Presentation of a stimulus is followed by an evoked response (traces *a* and *b*). A pair of stimuli result in a pair of evoked responses (trace *c*). If the subject is instructed to press a button as soon as the second stimulus is presented, the contingent negative variation emerges (trace *d*). Negativity is indicated by an upward deflection. (From Walter, Cooper, Aldridge, McCallum, and Winter 1964)

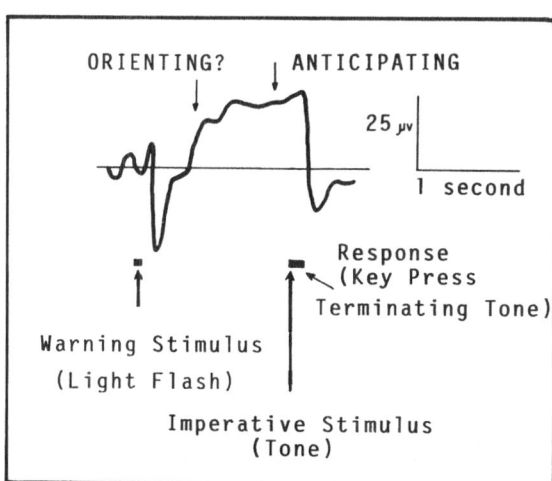

Fig. 2. Typical CNV, recorded during a short foreperiod. Negativity following the WS is assumed to reflect orienting; negativity preceding the RS is assumed to reflect anticipation or preparation for the response. Negativity is indicated by an upward deflection. (From Callaway 1975)

tween a central premotor CNV and a frontally dominant CNV, accompanying auditory discrimination. Weinberg and Papakostopoulos (1976) found differences in form and amplitude between frontal CNVs and those recorded at the vertex and the central and parietal electrode positions. The authors suggested that these differences might indeed reflect different functions of the cerebral sites involved in the information processing. To Callaway (1975) the results of many CNV experiments seemed to indicate two major processes: orienting and anticipation. The negativity following the WS would be related to orienting, the negativity at the end of the foreperiod to anticipation or preparation for the response (see Fig. 2). Such an interpretation is supported by findings during larger foreperiods, as will be shown in the next paragraph.

The Use of Larger Foreperiods

Connor and Lang (1969) and Lacey and Lacey (1970), using larger foreperiods than the traditional 1-s length, found a negative peak within 1 s after the WS and a negativity increasing to the moment the RS was going to be presented. Weerts and Lang (1973) called these waves the orienting response (OR) and the anticipatory response (AR): the same subdivision that was suggested later by Callaway (1975) also for the 1-s foreperiod slow waves (see Fig. 2).

Loveless and Sanford (1974a) related CNV more explicitly to the RT literature. They pointed to the predictable effects of varying foreperiod length on RT. Time uncertainty effects can be demonstrated by using foreperiods of different length, presented to the subjects in a regular or irregular way. In the regular condition the length is predictable within a block of trials; in the irregular condition it changes from trial to trial. If the foreperiod is varied over a number of seconds, in an irregular condition, a slow wave is always present at the start of the foreperiod, peaking within 1 s after the WS. Its time course is constant, regardless of foreperiod length. Therefore, the authors concluded that the slow wave was an effect of the WS. Indeed, the alerting properties of the WS (modality, intensity, and duration) influence its amplitude (Gaillard 1976; Klorman and Bentsen, 1975; Loveless 1975, 1976; Loveless and Sanford 1975; Rohrbaugh, Syndulko, and Lindsley 1976). After the disappearance of the slow wave no other slow potential was found in the irregular condition. However, if time uncertainty is minimal, i.e., in the regular condition, a second negative wave emerges. This is illustrated in the upper two traces of Fig. 3.

Loveless (1976) states that the second component of the CNV is related to the future movement. Arguments in favor of this interpretation stem from another study (Loveless and Sanford 1974b). Using fixed foreperiods of 4 s, Loveless and Sanford (1974b) gave two different instructions to their subjects: "motor" instructions, encouraging response speed, and "sensory" instructions, encouraging accuracy through careful attention to the RS. The early wave was not influenced by the instructions, but the late wave was: its amplitude varied with the RT, which was of course shorter under speed than under accuracy in-

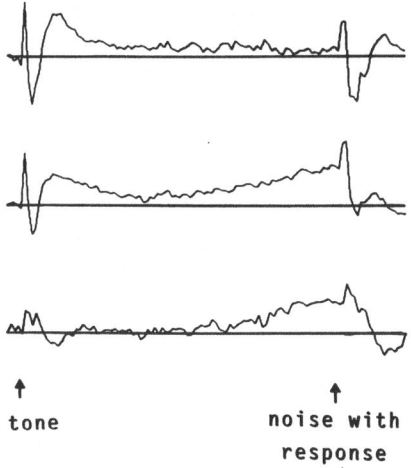

Fig. 3. CNV recorded during a 6-sec foreperiod in an irrecular (*top*) and a regular (*middle*) condition. A slow wave after the WS is present in the regular condition, i.e., when the subject's time uncertainty is rather small. Subtraction of both waves shows an RP (*bottom*). Negativity is indicated by an upward deflection. (From "Event related slow potentials of the brain as expressions of orienting functions" by Loveless N.E. in H. D. Kimmel, E. H. van Olst, and J. F. Orlebeke (Eds.) *The orienting reflex in humans,* 1979, 77–100. Copyright 1979 by Lawrence Erlbaum Associates Inc. Reprinted by permission)

tone   noise with
                                  response

structions. Besides the differences in functional properties, a difference in potential distribution was found. The early wave showed larger amplitudes over the frontal areas, the late wave over the central and parietal sites. This potential distribution has been corroborated by a number of authors. Rohrbaugh et al. (1976) demonstrated that the early and late wave showed the same topography as, respectively, the orienting potential evoked by a nonsignal stimulus and the premovement readiness potential (RP). Moreover, both the early wave and the orienting potential showed no hemisphere difference, whereas the late wave and the RP showed a comparable asymmetry, with larger amplitudes over the hemisphere contralateral to the movement side. The authors argued, therefore, that the summation of the early and late wave during a short foreperiod of 1 s might constitute the "classic" CNV. Gaillard (1976), who compared the topography of slow waves in 1- and 3-s foreperiods, came to a similar conclusion. Using a principal component analysis of the CNV during a 1-s foreperiod, Donchin, Kutas, and McCarthy (1977) found a frontal wave peaking at 475 ms and a central wave peaking at the time of the response. The latter results show that a long foreperiod is not a prerequisite to demonstrate the existence of two different slow waves.

Summarizing, we may conclude that the CNV consists of at least two components: an early wave, related to orienting, and a late wave, related to the future movements. In the next paragraph we will consider potentials related to preparation and execution of voluntary movements.

Movement-Related Potentials

Shortly after the first description of the CNV was published, Kornhuber and Deecke (1965) and Gilden, Vaughan, and Costa (1966) found another slow-wave complex in the EEG. This time it concerned a reflection of brain activity preceding a voluntary movement, e.g., pressing a button by finger flexion. In Fig. 4 the different components of what the latter authors termed "motor potential" are indicated by symbols: N_1, P_1, N_2, and P_2. They represent the successive negative and positive shifts, without a functional interpretation. The former authors used the following descriptive terms for the same components, respectively: *Bereitschaftspotential* (BP) or readiness potential (RP), premotion positivity (PMP), motor potential (MP), and reafferent potential (RAP). The time relation to the movement and the topographical distribution were described by Deecke and Kornhuber (1977) as follows. The RP is a bilateral, slowly increasing negative wave which appears at the anterior parietal and precentral electrodes. It starts about 800 ms prior to a brisk finger movement and is in the beginning symmetrical over both hemispheres. From 400 ms on it becomes asymmetrical, with larger amplitudes over the hemisphere contralateral to the movement side. At 150 ms prior to EMG onset, the hemisphere difference is significant. The PMP is bilateral and widespread, beginning about 90 ms prior to EMG onset. It is not present in all subjects. Its amplitude over the ipsilateral hemisphere is larger at parietal than at precentral recording sites. The MP is a unilateral wave. It starts 50 ms prior to EMG onset and is maximal over the hand area in the motor cortex. The authors suggest that the PMP reflects the actual command for the movements, whereas the MP corresponds to the motor cortex outflow. The RAP is a post-movement slow-wave complex, which is also present after passive movements and which seems to be related to proprioceptive reafferent activity.

There has been discussion about the time relation of the MP to the movement onset. Contrary to the findings of Deecke and Kornhuber, Gerbrandt, Goff, and Smith (1973) recorded a small negative wave 20–50 ms after the beginning of the

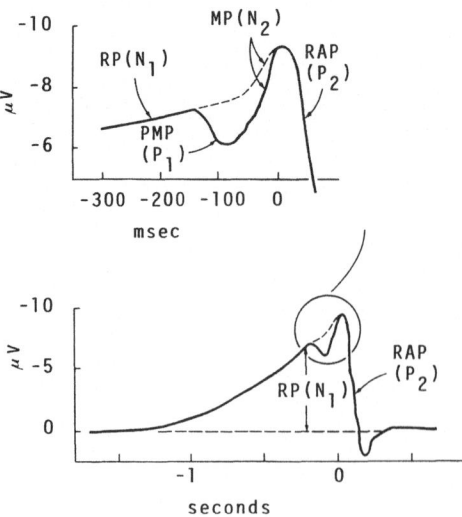

Fig. 4. Movement-related potentials. N_1 or readiness potential, N_2 or motor potential, P_1 or premotion positivity, and P_2 or reafferent potential. The *insert* shows the smaller P_1 and N_2 component which occur just prior to the movement (time zero). (From McAdam 1974)

movement over the frontal area with the same potential distribution as the so-matosensory evoked response. This led these authors to the conclusion that it was a reafferent potential. It is now generally accepted that both groups of authors are right and that indeed there is a premovement N_2 (or MP), whereas another small negative wave is present in the reafferent potential complex, which, for the time being, is called N_3 (Gerbrandt 1977). In recent studies aimed at the question of how many components can be distinguished in movement-related potentials, Shibasaki, Barret, Halliday, and Halliday (1980, 1981) described the following eight components:

1. A BP, increasing gradually from 1.5 or 1 s to about 500 ms prior to EMG onset. The onset of the BP is at the vertex; it shows a wide symmetrical distribution from frontal to parietal sites, its maximum being at the midline precentral-parietal region.
2. NS, a negative shift which is present from 500 to 90 ms prior to EMG onset. The gradient increases asymmetrically with contralateral larger amplitudes which are maximal over the precentral area. It also is present over the parietal, but not over the frontal, area.
3. $\overline{\text{P-50}}^1$, a small positive wave following the preceding negative peak. It shows a wide distribution over the precentral and parietal regions but predominantly over the ipsilateral hemisphere. In the precentral region the peak is followed by a negative wave, in the parietal region by another positive wave with an in-termediate negative inflexion.
4. $\overline{\text{N-10}}$, a sharp negative peak which is localized over the precentral area con-tralateral to the movement. This site corresponds to the projection area of the hand.
5. $\overline{\text{N+50}}$, a negative wave emerging bilaterally over the frontal region, after the EMG peak. There is a slight contralateral preponderance with finger move-ments.
6. $\overline{\text{P+90}}$, following the peak of N-10; this positive peak is found over the parietal and precentral region, contralateral to the movement side, although it is also present ipsilaterally.
7. $\overline{\text{N+160}}$: contralateral to the movement, the P+90 is followed by this negative wave, which is predominant over the parietal area.
8. $\overline{\text{P+300}}$: contralateral to the movement side of the finger, this wave is maximal over the precentral region, halfway between the vertex and the hand motor area.

Analysis of the significance of these different components is not possible with-out animal experiments. Before discussing some experiments with higher animals

---

[1] The horizontal bar used in designating this and the following components indicates that theoretically distinguishable components are described, of which the latency might vary in different experiments (Donchin, Callaway, Cooper, Desmedt, Goff, Hillyard, and Sutton 1977).

we will first draw attention to the fact that the CNV late wave and the RP seem very much alike. In the next section the question to what extent the CNV late wave is indeed identical to the RP will be examined. For a complete review we refer to Tecce and Cattanach (1982) and to Rohrbaugh and Gaillard (1983).

A Relation Between Contingent Negative Variation and Readiness Potential

McAdam, Knott, and Rebert (1969) were the first to realize that the anticipatory potential recorded during larger foreperiods had a morphology similar to the RP. Although CNV and RP are recorded under different experimental conditions, a voluntary movement has to be made in both paradigms. It could, therefore, be hypothesized that the similarity between CNV and RP is primarily based on the contribution of the motor system. Above, we discussed an experiment carried out by Loveless (1979), who recorded slow waves during foreperiods of different lengths. In the regular condition all foreperiods in a block had the same length, so that the subject could prepare for the moment the RS showed up and for the response to be given. In the irregular condition blocks consisted of foreperiods of different lengths, making such preparation improbable. In the first condition two waves were present, in the second only one (see Fig. 3). Loveless (1979) pointed out the fact that subtracting the first from the second curve results in an RP- like potential (Fig. 3, trace 3). Although he was of the opinion that the CNV late wave is an RP, several differences between CNV and RP have been put forward by Deecke and Kornhuber (1977). The CNV mostly shows a symmetrical distri- bution over both hemispheres, whereas the RP is larger over the hemisphere con- tralateral to the movement side. Moreover, the potential distribution in the an- terior- posterior axis seems to be different for both slow waves, the CNV am- plitudes being larger in the frontal area, while the RP amplitudes are larger over the central and parietal sites. RP amplitudes are usually smaller than CNV am- plitudes, their form being different in that the CNV increases more suddenly than the RP. Moreover, it has been argued that CNVs can be recorded during both short and long foreperiods, even when no immediate motor response was required from the subjects (Donchin, Gerbrandt, Leifer, and Tucker 1972; Lang, Öhman, and Simons 1978).

Arguments in favor of a motor interpretation of the CNV late wave stem largely from experiments in which larger foreperiods are used. In a recent review Rohrbaugh and Gaillard (1983) summarize the arguments as follows:

1. When no motor response is required, the CNV is attenuated during short fore- periods (Järvilehto and Frühstorfer 1970) and the terminal CNV is attenuated or absent during long foreperiods (Loveless 1975; Lang, Öhmann and Simons 1978; Gaillard 1980, see Fig. 5).
2. The terminal CNV is affected by task variables such as foreperiod duration, foreperiod variability, and response probability. In RT studies these factors have been assumed to affect the level of motor preparation (Niemi and Nää- tänen 1981).

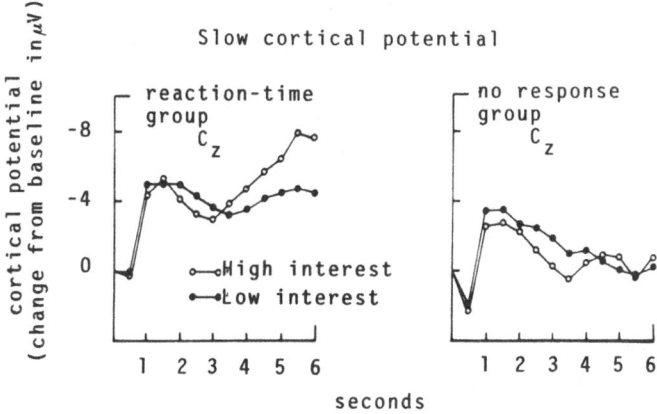

Fig. 5. Cortical slow waves as a function of response requirements (reaction time versus no response group) and the content of a slide presented as S_2 (high versus low interest). Foreperiod duration is 6 s. (From Lang, Öhman, and Simons 1978)

3. The amplitude of the terminal CNV is not increased preceding difficult discriminations as compared with easy ones, nor in RT tasks, nor in signal detection tasks (Perdok and Gaillard 1979).

4. Larger CNV amplitudes are found when more muscular effort is required for a response to S_2 (Low and McSherry 1968; Rebert, McAdam, Knott, and Irwin 1976). A similar result has been described for the RP (Kutas and Donchin 1977).

5. The amplitude of the terminal CNV is enhanced under speed instructions (Loveless and Sanford 1974b; Gaillard, Perdok and Varey 1980) and prior to fast responses when they are compared with slow responses from the same series (Rohrbaugh et al. 1976; Brunia and Vingerhoets 1980, see Fig. 6).

6. Terminal CNV and RP show the same left–right asymmetry preceding movements of the finger (Rohrbaugh et al. 1976) and of the foot (Brunia and Vingerhoets 1980; Brunia and Van den Bosch 1984), respectively. Prior to finger movements the CNV late wave and the RP show larger amplitudes over the hemisphere contralateral to the movement side, whereas prior to foot movements amplitudes are larger over the ipsilateral hemisphere. For an elaboration on this opposite hemisphere distribution, see Brunia and Van den Bosch (1984).

In spite of the ample evidence for the CNV late wave being an RP there remain obstacles to overcome. If RP and CNV late wave are recorded in one and the same experiment, both slow waves seem to be different in amplitude. The first experiment of this kind was done by Deecke, Becker, Grözinger, and Kriebel (1976). Subjects were asked to make a voluntary movement, followed, after a fixed interval, by an RS upon which the same movement had to be made again.

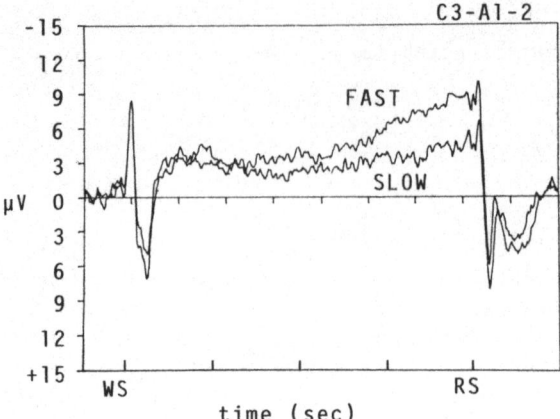

Fig. 6. CNV magnitude as a function of fast versus slow responses during a 4-s foreperiod. A plantar flexion of the right foot served as the response. (From Brunia and Vingerhoets 1980)

A similar experiment was done by McCallum (1978). Both experiments were primarily done to demonstrate a different potential distribution for CNV and RP. The interval, however, was short, i.e., 1.5 s. McCallum (1978) reported amplitudes of CNV being larger than of RP at frontal, central, and parietal electrode positions.

To allow for a better development of a CNV late wave Brunia and Vingerhoets (1981) carried out an RP-CNV study with a 4-s interval, a plantar flexion of the foot being the response. The CNV late wave was larger than the RP, in accordance with McCallum's data. These data suggest that the CNV late wave is an RP superimposed on another negativity, which itself might be related to certain non-motor aspects of the RT experiment. There is, however, another possibility. Gaillard (1980) investigated slow potentials and EMGs preceding a finger flexion in four different conditions. Subjects were asked to make a voluntary movement every 6–7 s. Afterwards, they were asked to perform an RT task with a fixed foreperiod of 4 s. Next, they had to perform a synchronization task, in which they tried to press a button as near to 4 s after the WS as possible. Finally, they were involved in a detection task in which they had to indicate with a delayed response whether the RS was presented 4 s after the WS or 500–600 ms later. The CNV late wave was largest in the RT task, but so was the EMG activity. Rohrbaugh, Varner, and Ellison (Rohrbaugh and Gaillard 1983) also found larger EMG activity in agonist muscles in an RT task as compared with a voluntary movement. These data suggest that the motor outputs in a warned RT task and a voluntary movement are different and that this difference could be related to a difference in amplitude of CNV late wave and RP. In other words, the extra negativity upon which the smaller RP is superimposed might also be a motor-related negativity. In their simultaneous recording of EEG and EMG activity, Brunia and Vingerhoets (1980) found a systematic increase of mean EMG activity in their subjects during a fixed 4-s foreperiod. The response was a plantar flexion of the right foot. Parallel to a larger mean CNV late wave preceding fast responses they also found a steeper increase in mean EMG activity. This suggests a common factor influencing the EEG, EMG, and RT. However, the results were not analyzed on an individual basis.

To meet this objection a new experiment was done (Haagh and Brunia, in press) in which bilateral EMG activity was recorded from both calf muscles during a 4-s foreperiod, together with EEG activity. The response was again a plantar flexion of the right foot. Subjects were divided post hoc into two groups: one with distinct EMG activity during the foreperiod, the other with no EMG activity. Mean CNV early wave and N_1 amplitude were larger when EMG activity was present than without EMG activity but there was no relation to RT, thus indicating a dissociation between performance on the one hand and EMG and EEG on the other hand. However, larger CNV late wave amplitudes were found prior to fast RTs as compared with slow RTs; this increase in late wave amplitude was unrelated to agonist EMG level during the foreperiod. At this moment we assume that these recent findings exemplify the existence of at least two different functional attributions to the late wave. The first might be a general way of preparation for the response; the other is related to response speed. The assumption of the generality of the first process was supported by the fact that muscle-tension-related negativity was already present during the CNV early wave and even in the N_1 component following the WS, i.e., before the onset of the increment of agonist EMG.

Summarizing, the CNV late wave and the RP give similar results to the extent that the functional demands of RP and RT tasks are identical. It is obvious that at least part of the preparatory processes in an RT task are not unique to movement preparation. It would be of great help if the sources of the slow potentials and their respective contributions in different tasks were better known. It is therefore now advantageous to discuss some relevant findings from the animal literature.

Possible Sources

From the foregoing it has become evident that the interpretation of changes in slow waves and their relation to psychophysiological processes is very difficult. If one is also interested in the brain structures relevant for these processes, the situation becomes even more complicated. One of the difficulties with slow waves in humans is that the source they stem from is unknown. It is possible to record systematic EEG changes on the scalp that, originating from the brain stem, arrive at the skin by means of volume conduction. In other words the scalp recordings reflect not only local activity from the cortex underneath, but also from deeper structures in the brain. Moreover, skin, skull, and meninges have different conduction characteristics, influencing the potential amplitude and distribution. For these and other reasons it is difficult to be sure about the localization of the source of the electrophysiological activity one is interested in. Within certain limits animal experiments can be helpful, since electrodes can be placed directly in the cortex and in subcortical structures.

As far as surface negative slow potentials are concerned, Caspers, Speckmann, and Lehmenkühler (1980) concluded that neuronal elements in the upper layers of the cortex play a dominant role in their generation. Especially dendritic potentials seem to contribute to them, whereas in the deeper cortical layers changes in cell membrane potential are of importance. If slow potentials are recorded transcortically by a pair of electrodes, one almost at the surface and the other some millimeters deeper, it may happen that a negative wave is recorded at the surface and a positive one at depth. Such a polarity reversal indicates that the generator is situated between both electrodes (Wood and Allison 1981; see Fig. 7). On the basis of histological knowledge of the cortex it can be tentatively concluded which cell structures are involved in the function one is investigating.

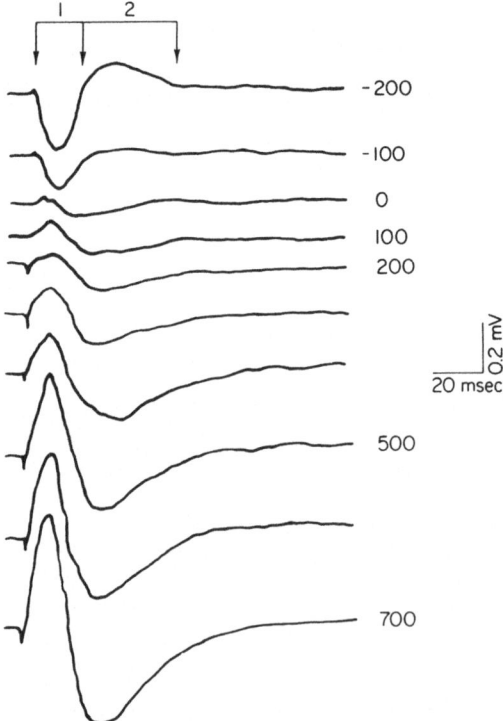

Fig. 7. Polarity reversal of extracellular potentials recorded at different depths in cat prepyriform cortex. Depths are in micrometers while negativity is indicated by a downward deflection. (From Biedenbach and Stevens 1969)

Animal experiments have another advantage. The activity of single cells or multiple units can be recorded in comparable experiments as done in humans (Evarts 1981). Performance-related changes in firing pattern of groups of cells at a certain level of the cortex give a more direct picture of the relevant structures than do slow potentials. The gap between recordings of single-cell activity and of slow potentials can be filled by recording multiple unit activity and slow waves simultaneously as we will see in the next paragraphs. There we will draw attention to animal CNV and RP studies, in order to appreciate which brain structures these slow potentials might come from.

Animal Contingent Negative Variation Studies

Slow potentials during a warned RT experiment have been recorded in animal studies in different subcortical structures and in the cortex (Rebert 1972). CNV-like slow waves, especially in the frontal cortex of monkeys, have been described in a number of papers (Low et al. 1966; Borda 1970; Donchin, Otto, Gerbrandt and Pribram 1971; Hablitz 1973).

As far as subcortical structures are concerned, Rebert (1977) considered the slow potentials he recorded as reflecting local events, not as volume-conducted potentials from remote generators, since in different subcortical areas slow-positive and slow-negative potentials were present simultaneously. Subcortically generated slow-negative potentials were supposed to reflect an increment in neuronal activity, whereas the positive slow potentials would be related to a decrease in neuronal activity (Rebert 1973). In the mesencephalic reticular formation slow-negative waves were found, whereas in the caudate nucleus a slow-positive wave was present (Fig. 8, Rebert 1977). The distribution of slow waves which are present simultaneously at different locations during the foreperiod of an RT experiment suggests the existence of a network of structures that play an active role in the information processing under study. In this respect it is important that McCallum, Papakostopoulos, Gombi, Winter, Cooper, and Griffith (1973) have recorded in man positive event-related slow potentials in or near the caudate nucleus and negative ones in the reticular formation, similar to Rebert's (1977) findings in monkeys. Such results suggest that, all circumstances being equal, comparable processes take place at homologous sites in the monkey and human brain, irrespective of the anatomical differences between both. In other words, under certain conditions the generalization from monkey to man seems to be warranted.

Evidence for a cortical origin stems among others from the work of Borda (1970), who recorded EEG activity in the monkey during a conditioning process. The animal learned to wait after a click until a tone was presented 1 s later, upon which a lever had to be pressed. Borda (1970) found two different and independent cortical slow waves during the waiting period. The first, recorded approximately precentrally, was more variable as conditioning continued and seemed to be related to arousal. The second was found in the frontal area, per-

PAIRED TONE

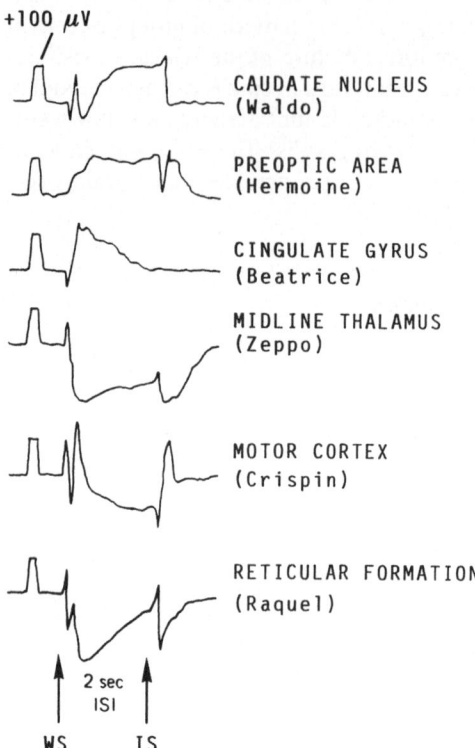

Fig. 8. Examples of slow potentials recorded in several brain regions of macaques during a simple RT task (*WS*, warning stimulus; *IS*, imperative stimulus). (From Rebert 1972)

sisted during overtraining, and was supposed to be related to the CNV. In a later paper McSherry, Borda, and Hablitz (1977) have pointed out the rather generalized activation of the cortex in the beginning of the conditioning process. The authors suggested that, once the relationship between S1 and S2 has been established, only those areas in the cortex which are specifically related to the perception of the stimuli and the execution of the response need to be primed. In the monkey this seems to be Brodmann's area 6 and the more frontally localized region of the sulcus principalis, known to be of importance for the information storage in delayed response tasks (Gross and Weiskrantz 1964).

Delayed response and RT paradigms are very much alike. In the former a cue signal is presented, which after a delay interval has to be followed by a choice, contingent upon the cue. In the former paragraph it was mentioned that slow potentials and single-unit activity can be recorded under almost identical circumstances. If systematic changes are found in both, this suggests a causal relationship or a common factor behind both as we will see now.

During delayed response tasks slow potentials have been recorded from the prefrontal cortex around the sulcus principalis. One of them starts at the end of the presentation of the cue and reaches its maximum at the beginning of the delay (Stamm and Rosen 1973). Fuster and Alexander (1971) found an increase in single-unit activity in the prefrontal cortex during the delay as can be seen in Fig. 9. They demonstrated that this increased activity was only present after the animals were trained to give the appropriate response. Thus the critical factor was an established contingency between cue and response. Later, Fuster (1981) suggested that the source of the CNV or one of its components might be this prefrontal neuron population.

Consequences for the Human Contingent Negative Variation

The frontal lobe in man is also related to delayed response tasks (Milner 1974), and its role in the orienting response is beyond doubt (e.g., Luria and Homskaya 1970). In view of the fact that in longer foreperiods at least two CNV components are present, we are inclined to think that the early wave might be the result of activity in comparable neuron populations in the prefrontal cortex as has been described by Fuster and Alexander (1971). The activity in these areas could be related to a mnemonic process of retaining the cue or a setting for the forthcoming response, as Fuster (1981) has suggested. However, the present authors think that the latter function is realized more specifically by another part of the frontal lobe: the premotor cortex, as was suggested by McSherry et al. (1977). More evidence for this point of view is put forward in the next paragraph.

Animal Movement-Related Potentials

Arezzo and Vaughan (1975) studied slow potential shifts in the monkey brain related to wrist extension movements. They pointed out the similar morphology of the movement-related potentials in monkey and man. They found three pre-EMG onset components: N_1, P_1, and N_2. The distribution of N_1 was "roughly comparable to N_2," and P_1 was not systematically present in contrast to N_2, which started about 90 ms before EMG onset and reached its maximum over the contralateral precentral gyrus. Two post-EMG onset potentials were found: P_2 and P_3 (see Fig. 10). P_2 was found above the pre- and post-central cortex, and dominated contralaterally, in contrast to the bilaterally symmetrical P_3. A reversal in polarity within the cortex indicated the site of the source: N_2 was restricted to the hand area over the precentral gyrus, P_2 to the pre- and postcentral gyrus, and P_3 to area 5.

In later papers, Arezzo, Vaughan, and Koss (1977) and Arezzo and Vaughan (1980) recorded, besides slow waves, multiple-unit activity (MUA) in the cortex. Thus it became possible to localize the sources more accurately. N_2 showed the polarity reversal at the same level as that where MUA was found to be maximal (lamina 5). The transcortical reversal of P_2 was more superficial, in agreement with the presence of MUA in the more superficial layers. Concurrent with the P_3

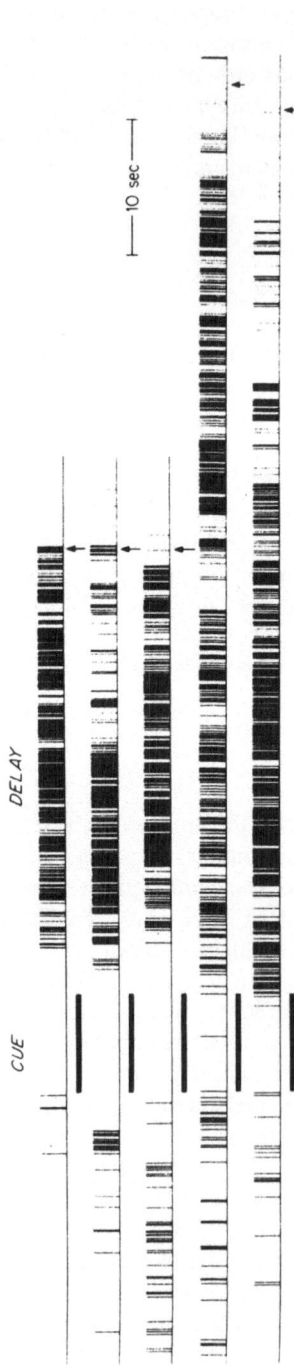

Fig. 9. Single unit activity in prefrontal cortex of the monkey, during five delayed response trials. Increased activation of single units is observed even during delays of 1 min. Firing returns to normal when the monkey responds (see *arrows*). (From Fuster and Alexander 1971)

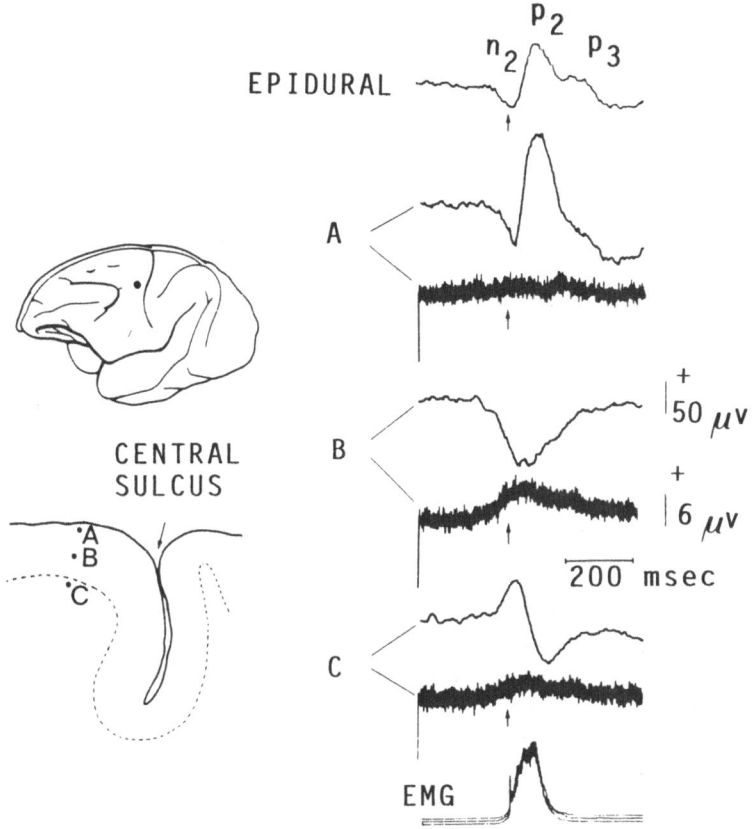

Fig. 10. Movement-related slow potentials and averaged multiple unit activity recorded at three levels within the posterior portion of the precentral gyrus in the monkey. *At the bottom of the panel* the averaged EMGs from each series are shown. Potentials were recorded contralateral to the movement side. (From Arezzo, Vaughan, and Koss 1977)

potential reversal, MUA was only found postcentrally. It should be noted that in these studies slow-positive potential components were accompanied by an increase in MUA, in contrast to what Rebert (1973) had found in subcortical nuclei. Recently, Arezzo and Vaughan (1980) refined their original description of N_2 and P_2 by distinguishing N_{2a}, N_{2b}, P_{2a}, and P_{2b}. A polarity reversal was found with N_{2a} and P_{2b} (lamina 5 and lamina 2–3, respectively). N_{2a} was supposed to reflect the corticospinal outflow inducing the start of the movement. P_{2b} could represent the corollary discharges or efferent copies from cortical and subcortical structures, in other words: feedback activity from central structures involved in the execution of the movement. The N_{2b}–P_{2a} complex was supposed to reflect short latency reafferent activity within the cortex around the central sulcus.

Gemba, Sasaki, and Hashimoto (1980) also recorded slow potentials in the monkey brain preceding a wrist extension. They found a symmetrical potential distribution in the premotor cortex, in contrast to the motor cortex, which showed larger amplitudes contralateral to the movement side. A transcortical polarity reversal was found only in the contralateral premotor and motor cortex (Hashimoto, Gemba, and Sasaki 1979). Comparison of slow potentials prior to hand and to foot movements showed that the polarity reversal was restricted to the hand and foot area, respectively, although prior to foot movements potentials were more widespread. Thus, again a contralateral source of the premovement potentials was found, whereas at the same time the bilateral involvement of the premotor cortex was suggested. Accepting the argument that the similarity in morphology of slow potentials in monkey and man suggests a comparable involvement of the homologous cortical structures, we will see next what preliminary conclusions might be drawn from this for the human movement-related potentials.

Consequences for the Human Movement-Related Potentials

Although many questions remain to be answered, the comparison of animal results with the carefully described slow potential components in man initiates an understanding of the localization of the sources of the different components. For the research in monkeys the combined recording of slow waves and MUA has been demonstrated to be useful. Progress in the research of slow potentials in man can be made only by using a large number of electrodes to allow for a simultaneous recording from as many places as possible. Whereas some clarity develops about the localization of the sources, their functional role is still far from clear.

To indicate but one problem: the largest of the movement-related potentials, the RP, is present not only over the precentral gyrus, but also over the premotor cortex. A combined recording of slow potentials and MUA from the premotor cortex has not yet been done. However, separate recordings of both have been published. Preceding self-paced hand movements, slow potentials have been recorded in the motor and premotor cortex of monkeys by Hashimoto, Gemba, and Sasaki (1980). The size of the potentials in the motor and premotor cortex changed more or less as a function of the change in load (see Fig. 11). The authors suggested that the potentials might represent a central preparation process for the movement, as a consequence of the animal's estimation of the force required. They further suggested that the premotor cortex showed the preparatory activity at an earlier point in time than the motor cortex. Therefore, Hashimoto et al. (1980) concluded that the motor cortex was more closely related to the execution of the movement, the premotor cortex playing a role in the motor programming.

Tanji, Taniguchi, and Saga (1980) have shown that activity in neurons in the supplementary motor area (SMA) is instruction dependent. The altered discharge

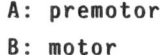
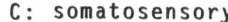

A: premotor

B: motor

C: somatosensory

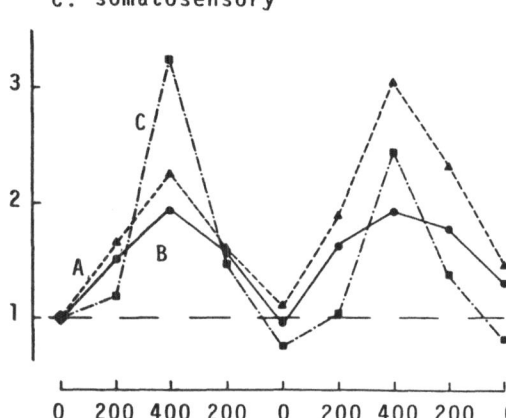

Fig. 11. Relation between magnitude of premovement slow potentials and load of the response. Recordings were made from the premotor, motor, and somatosensory cortex. *Abscissa,* magnitude of load in grams. *Ordinate,* ratio between areas of the premovement potentials during load and during the first no-load session. (From Hashimoto, Gemba, and Sasaki 1980)

activity did not cause EMG changes, suggesting that no matter which neurons were activated the spinal motoneurons were not excited above their firing threshold. The authors suggested that SMA neurons were also active prior to those in the motor cortex. They cited a number of papers, showing connections from SMA to striatum, thalamus, pontine nuclei, red nucleus, and spinal cord. These efferent connections could provide the neural basis for the development of the prepared responsiveness. This could go along with subliminal changes in the excitability of the motoneurons toward their firing threshold. Arguments for this assumption are provided by reflex studies in man, as will be shown later on.

The bilateral presence of the RP has been a reason to argue that preparation for a movement involves both hemispheres (Kornhuber 1974), the execution being restricted to the motor cortex contralateral to the movement sides. This has consequences for the interpretation of CNV studies. During the foreperiod of RT experiments two slow waves are generally found, an early one related to the WS and a later one related to the movement. We now have to face the problem that the latter presumably does not represent the activity of only one generator. On the contrary, it is plausible that the slow wave over the premotor cortex represents a process different from the ones recorded over the motor cortex and the parietal cortex.

It is a common finding in scalp EEG recordings in man that RP and CNV late waves are present over the parietal area. However, Gemba, Hashimoto, and Sasaki (1979), recording intracortical movement-related potentials in monkey, found hardly any RP in area 7 and no RP at all in area 19. Arezzo and Vaughan (1980) also found no activity in area 7 (see Fig. 12 for a localization of cortical areas in man). They reported that recordings posterior to the central sulcus never

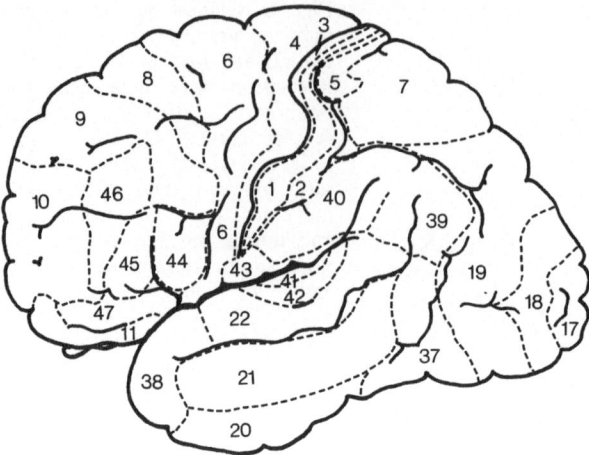

Fig. 12. Areas in the left hemisphere in man, classified according to Brodmann

revealed any slow potentials or MUA prior to movement onset. These results suggest that parietal RP and CNV late waves in man might point to volume-conducted activity rather than to a parietal source. A further argument in favor of the volume conduction interpretation would be the presence of an RP recorded over the skull above the parietal cortex in monkeys. However, such data are so far not available.

On the other hand, it is known that in the monkey a number of parietal neurons can be triggered by visual stimuli, but only when these stimuli play a role in some kind of movement to be performed (Hyvarinen and Poranen 1974). Lamarre, Spidalieri, Burby, and Lund (1980) reported the existence of neurons in the depth of the parietal sulcus which were activated 100 msec after a light signal in the contralateral visual field prior to an arm movement. These findings suggest that cells in the parietal cortex function as an interface between the sensory and motor system and that their function in the information processing is earlier in time than that of the motor (and premotor?) cortex. Lamarre et al. (1980) hypothesized that the parietal cells, among other things, might play a role in the decision process as to whether or not to make a movement. Such cell groups could be even present in larger amounts in man, being one of the sources of the parietal CNV late wave. However, for the human RP such reasoning does not help since in that case there are no visual stimuli upon which a movement has to be made. One of the characteristics of RP studies is the timing of the voluntary movements, since they have to be made at not too short intervals. Central processes, related to the decision to make the movement, might perhaps also be reflected in the parietal RP. However probable that may be, it should be kept in mind that the similarity of RP and CNV late wave over the motor and parietal cortex might be rather misleading, since the underlying processes in both brain areas are presumably very different.

Another problem is the voluntary behavior during RT experiments. After all, how voluntary is a response produced after an RS? Of course the subject can refuse to follow the instructions, but once the constraints are accepted the subject's behavior is largely determined by the stimuli presented. Even with RP experiments such problems arise.

Recently a paper has been published concerning the differences in RP preceding spontaneous and preplanned voluntary acts (Libet, Wright and Gleason 1982). In most RP experiments subjects are asked to repeat a certain kind of movement over and over again with intervals of a few seconds. Moreover, they must try to prevent making eye movements or blinks, which cause artefacts in the EEG recordings. This is quite a different situation from the one in which spontaneous voluntary movements are made.

Libet et al. (1982) reasoned that RPs might also be different in both cases. They compared the slow potentials preceding the self-initiated voluntary acts and the preset motor acts. Three different RP types were found. Type I was a ramp-like wave, starting about 1000 ms before EMG onset. Type II started 700–400 ms prior to EMG onset, whereas the negativity of Type III did not start before 250 –200 ms. Preplanned RPs were mostly of Type I, whereas the spontaneous motor act was preceded by Type II or Type III. Type I resembled the RP as described by Deecke and Kornhuber (1977). Type II corresponds to the $\overline{\text{NS} \, (-500-90)}$ of Shibasaki et al. (1980) and thus to the asymmetrical component of Deecke and Kornhuber (1977). For Type III no clear counterpart in self-paced RPs was present.

The asymmetry of Type II suggests, according to the authors, a contribution from the motor cortex, as was also indicated by Arezzo and Vaughan (1980). However, Libet et al. (1982) stressed the fact that the potential is that large at the vertex that another source has to contribute to this slow wave too. Again the SMA could be a good candidate, although the authors are still hesitant to state that explicitly since direct recordings are not available. They suggest, however, the existence of two different processes. Process I is associated with the development of preparation to act in the near future (within some seconds), thus with time estimation. Process II is associated with voluntary choice and the more endogenous intention to act. It can be present in the absence of or in sequence with Process I.

Preliminary Conclusions

The foreperiod of an RT experiment starts with the presentation of a WS. It is known that the physical aspects of the stimulus are reflected in the early components of the evoked potential. These modality-specific electrophysiological changes are recorded in area 17 when a visual stimulus is used and in area 22 when a tone is presented to the subject (see Fig. 12). Psychological effects have been found as early as 200 ms after stimulus presentation, at least in certain experiments (Näätänen 1982).

Early psychological effects are also modality specific. A later component, the P300, seems to be related to the evaluation of the significance of the stimulus. It is not modality specific and its amplitude is maximal over the parietal cortex. This does not imply that its source is localized in the parietal lobe (Wood and Allison 1981). After the P300, negativity prevails over the cortex during the total length of the foreperiod. There are corticocortical connections between the secondary visual and auditory projection areas and the prefrontal cortex. It is not known whether they play a role in the succession of the different processes taking place during the foreperiod, but the next electrophysiological changes are found over the frontal cortex.

The early CNV wave is presumably related to orienting and mnemonic processes. One of its sources is situated in the human homologous area of the banks of the sulcus principalis in monkeys. The continuing negativity before the late wave starts perhaps indicates that another source is involved. The premotor cortex is activated next, perhaps via corticocortical connections from the prefrontal cortex. Its activity starts at an earlier moment than that of the motor cortex. Moreover the premotor cortex is activated bilaterally. The RP in this area presumably reflects the timing of the future response. Different subcortical, brain stem, and spinal motor structures are activated from the premotor cortex and the SMA. This might be part of a specific, but aselective, preparatory process. The motor cortex seems to be activated more than 1 s before the movement is going to be made. The asymmetrical RP ($\overline{\text{NS} -500-90}$) that can be recorded over the motor cortex seems to be part of a selective preparatory process, blending into the MP (N_2), which itself is a reflection of the final corticospinal outflow guiding the movement.

The Spinal Level

To execute a voluntary movement alpha motoneurons in the spinal cord have to be depolarized below a critical value at which they start firing. Preparation for a movement presumably also implies a depolarization but without reaching that critical value. In man it is impossible to record the changes in membrane potential of motoneurons in the spinal cord. An indirect method to estimate these changes, however, is available by means of evoking monosynaptic reflexes (Paillard 1955).

Monosynaptic Reflexes as a Tool

If a tap on the Achilles tendon is given, the calf muscle (musculus triceps surae) is stretched for a brief moment. The change in length is recorded by the annulospiral endings in the muscle spindle. They cause a depolarization of the agonist motoneurons via a monosynaptic connection of the I a afferent fibers, resulting in a contraction of the muscle. The electromyographic response, a triphasic compound action potential, can be recorded by means of surface electrodes attached to the skin over the agonist. Its peak-to-peak value is an indication of the number of motoneurons from the pool firing more or less simultaneously. If the impact of the eliciting stimulus is kept constant within a session, the variations in amplitude reflect, to a large extent, changes in excitability of the motoneurons, although presynaptic influences on the afferent fibers might also play a role (see Fig. 13 for a schematic representation of the reflex circuit).

A voluntary plantar flexion, i.e., an extension movement of the foot, is brought about by contraction of the calf muscles. The final common path for this

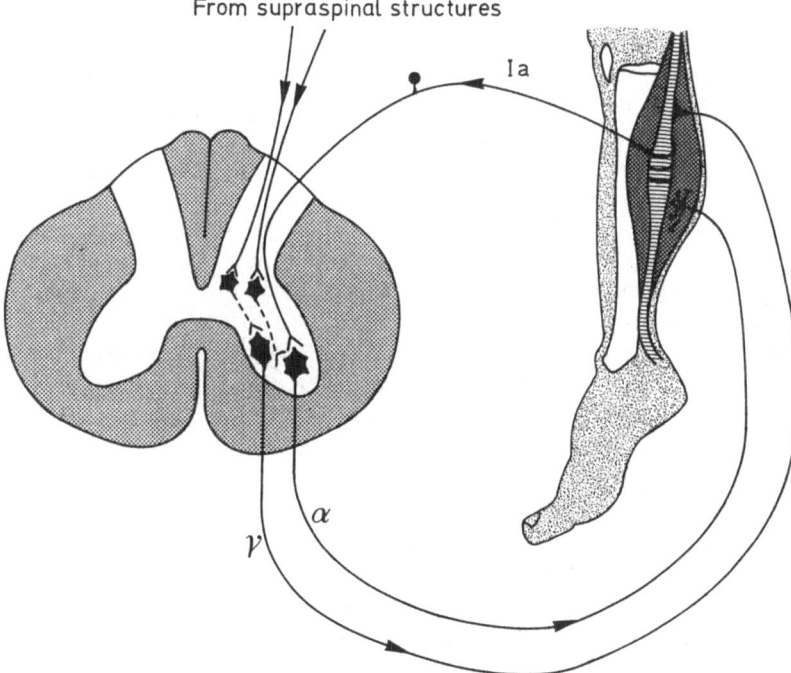

Fig. 13. Schematic representation of the reflex circuit showing the more important connections between the triceps surae muscle and the spinal cord as well as the way the gain of the reflex can be modulated by supraspinal influences. When the muscle is stretched the intrafusal fibers of the muscle spindles which lie in parallel to the extrafusal fibers are also stretched. (A muscle spindle is represented *lightly shaded* in the middle of the muscle.) This leads to an increased activity in the I a afferent fibers, which causes a depolarization of the alpha motoneurons. This, in turn, causes the muscle to contract. The gamma motoneurons play a role, as they innervate the muscle spindles. In this way, the muscle spindle's sensitivity to stretch can be preset. Facilitation of gamma and alpha motoneurons, however, mostly seems to be accomplished in a coactivated manner. Only descending influences on the reflex loop are shown in the Figure. Presynaptic inhibitory influences on the I a afferents as well as postsynaptic influences originating in other muscles, for instance, are omitted

movement and the Achilles tendon (T) reflex is the same. This makes the T reflex an interesting tool to estimate the changes in the excitability of the agonist motoneurons during the preparatory process. Moreover, the changes in excitability of motoneurons contralateral to the movement side can also be estimated by evoking the T reflexes bilaterally. Finally, a comparison of changes in T reflex amplitudes can be made preceding various kinds of movements, which are realized via motoneurons localized at different levels of the neuraxis. Thus, the various possibilities of using T reflexes during the foreperiods of RT experiments may contribute to an insight in the nature of preparatory processes. Hereafter, some experiments will be discussed which were done in our laboratory and which were aimed at unraveling the spinal preparatory processes which lead to response execution. These processes concern motoneurons that function sometimes as agonist and sometimes as antagonist, and that are sometimes uninvolved in the response. Depending on their functioning in the response execution we will see that selective and aselective aspects of the preparatory processes can be distinguished. The former concern the triceps motoneurons innervating the agonist; the latter the same motoneurons when they are not involved in the response.

The experiments are thus based on the following considerations.

1. If a unilateral plantar flexion of the foot is prepared and T reflexes are evoked simultaneously in both legs, the calf muscles ipsilateral to the movement side are involved in the response, whereas those contralateral to the movement side are not. The excitability of motoneurons of both involved and uninvolved muscles is tested. These motoneurons are localized at the same level of the spinal cord (the lumbosacral level).

2. If a unilateral finger movement is prepared and T reflexes are evoked simultaneously in both legs, neither calf muscle is involved in the response. The response is brought about via motoneurons in the cervical part of the spinal cord. Only the excitability of uninvolved motoneurons is tested, which are localized at a level different from the one at which the movement is carried out.

3. If a unilateral dorsiflexion, i.e., a flexion movement of one foot, is prepared, neither calf muscle is involved in the response. The excitability of only uninvolved motoneurons is tested in this situation. Note, however, that the motoneurons of the uninvolved calf muscle and the motoneurons of the agonist, i.e., the musculus tibialis anterior, are all localized at the lumbar level.

We will discuss changes in reflex amplitudes primarily from a motor viewpoint, i.e., we will treat them as part of electrophysiological processes that are related to the preparation for a response. From a pragmatic point of view preparatory processes are defined as aspecific and specific. Changes in the CNS which are not unique to preparation for a response are called aspecific. By specific changes we mean those processes that are necessary for the preparation of a movement. Specific changes may be aselective or selective. By aselective changes we mean those changes which are generalized throughout the CNS and can be observed prior to all kinds of movements. Selective changes, on the other hand, are not widespread but focussed. They are only observed in structures and muscles which are primarily involved in the movement.

In the reflex experiments to be described, a 4-s fixed foreperiod was employed, which was followed by intertrial intervals of 16 s. During these intertrial intervals reflexes were evoked, which served as a baseline level for the reflex amplitudes obtained at discrete points in time during the foreperiod.

Reflex Changes and Their Dependence upon a Motor Response

With the first three experiments our aim was to demonstrate that no changes in the excitability of motoneurons are present in case no overt motor response is prepared.

Reflex Changes During Passive Listening

In the first experiment, T reflexes were evoked at 100, 200, 2000, 3500, 3700, 3800, 3900, 4000, 4100, 4150, 4200, 4250, and 4300 ms after the WS. These were the same points in time as were used in most other experiments that will be discussed later. In these experiments characteristic indications of motor preparation were expected at the end of the foreperiod. Therefore most reflexes were evoked between 3500 and 4300 ms after the WS. As soon as subjects become aware of this, they might prepare for the arrival of the reflex, even if there is no response to give. Should that be the case then it could be expected that certain changes in amplitude might also show up if reflexes are evoked in an experiment in which no response is asked from the subject. In the present experiment S1 and S2 were tones, to assure that both stimuli were noticed by the subjects. No response was required; subjects were instructed to await quietly the end of the experiment in a relaxed state.

The results are shown in Fig. 14.

1. After the S1 a small increase in T-reflex amplitudes in both legs can be seen.
2. During the remainder of the interval between S1 and S2 reflex amplitudes in both legs are not different from the baseline.
3. After the S2 an increase in amplitude can be seen similar to that after the S1.

The peak recorded at 100 ms after the S1 cannot be related to preparation for a movement, since no response had to be given. During the remainder of the "foreperiod," amplitudes are not different from the baseline. Anticipation of the arrival of a reflex does not play a role or, if it does, it is not manifest in the T-reflex amplitudes. The peak after the S1 is of a similar size to that after the S2. Both stimuli had the same physical properties. Thus, presentation of a stimulus increases the reflex amplitude. That is, however, a very well known fact already described by Paillard (1955) and several others (Davis and Beaton 1968; Beale 1971; Rossignol and Melvill-Jones 1976). Such an increase may be part of an orienting response. It is not, under the present conditions, related to any motor preparation. The important outcome of this experiment is that possible antici-

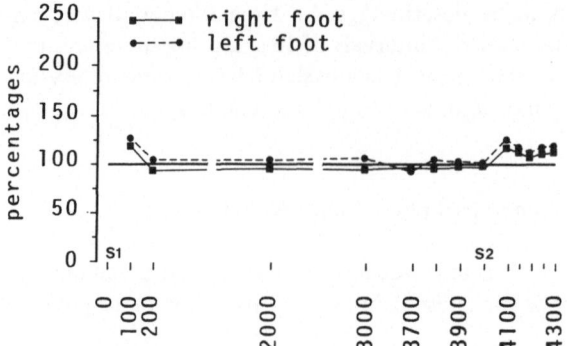

Fig. 14. Mean amplitudes of T reflexes evoked in both legs during and shortly after a fixed 4-s interval between two identical auditory stimuli. No task was required. *Baseline,* mean amplitude of reflexes evoked in the middle of 16-s intertrial intervals, calculated per subject. *Abscissa,* points in time of the reflex-eliciting stimulus. *Ordinate,* relative reflex amplitude. (From Brunia 1984)

pation effects which might be caused by the used points in time distribution are not reflected in the amplitude of the T reflex.

Reflex Changes During Stimulus Anticipation

In the second experiment (Scheirs and Brunia, in press) subjects were involved in a guessing task. The WS at 0 ms was again a tone and the S2 at 4000 ms a light that could show up on either the left or the right side. Subjects had to indicate on which side they expected the arrival of the S2 by pressing a button in one of the chair arms. The movement had to be made some seconds in advance of the WS on the same side as the S2 was expected. Subjects were rewarded for correct predictions. Since no response had to be prepared during the foreperiod, no changes in T-reflex amplitudes were expected. As can be seen in Fig. 15, no other systematic changes in amplitude are present between the WS and the S2 than the peaks following the WS and the S2. Therefore it can be concluded that the expectancy of a significant stimulus to come does not alter reflex amplitudes either.

Reflex Changes Prior to a Delayed Response

In the third experiment (Brunia, Damen, and Van Dieren, in preparation) subjects had to postpone their responses until 1–2 s after the presentation of the RS. Since there was no pressure for fast responding, motor preparation was supposed to be low or absent. The results are depicted in Fig. 16. Apart from a small in-

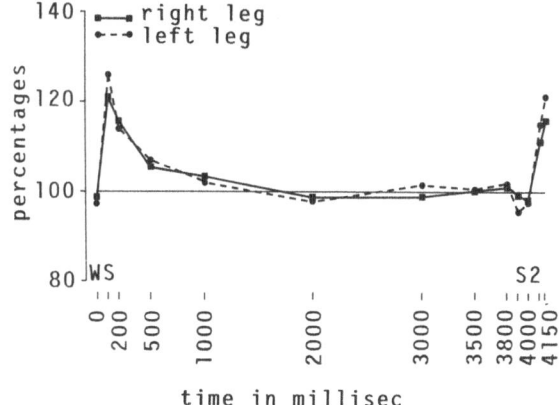

Fig. 15. Achilles tendon reflex amplitudes during stimulus anticipation. The subject's task was to make a prediction about the occurrence of S2 on the left or on the right side by pressing a key prior to presentation of the WS. No other motor response than the key press was required. See also legends to Figure 14. (From Scheirs and Brunia, in press)

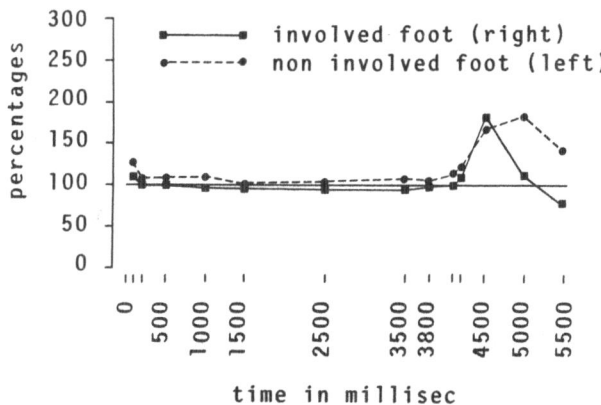

Fig. 16. Mean amplitudes of T reflexes, evoked in both legs during and after a fixed 4-s foreperiod of a simple RT experiment. In this condition the subjects had to postpone their response. See also legends to Figure 14. (From Brunia, Damen, and Van Dieren, in preparation)

crease after the WS, amplitudes again showed no changes from the baseline during the foreperiod.

Summarizing the results of the first three experiments, it can be concluded that neither the expectancy of a reflex to be evoked nor the expectancy of a stimulus to come influences the excitability of the motoneurons. When there is no time stress to give a response, there are no changes in reflex amplitudes either.

In the experiments to be discussed next, we will demonstrate that there are systematic changes in reflex amplitudes which might reflect motor preparation.

Reflex Changes Prior to Foot and Finger Movements

The considerations upon which this experiment was based were described on page 57. Four response conditions were studied. After the presentation of the RS a plantar flexion on the left or right side had to be made in Conditions A and B, respectively. A flexion of the index finger on the left or right side was the response in Conditions C and D, respectively (Brunia, Scheirs, and Haagh 1982). Reflexes were evoked at the same points in time as in the first experiment. The results are shown in Fig. 17.

The results show a clear difference with those of the first three experiments.

1. A bilateral increase in amplitude is found 200 ms after the WS in all conditions.
2. During the remainder of the foreperiod a difference between finger and foot response conditions is present. Preceding finger movement amplitudes on both sides are larger than the baseline. Prior to a foot response reflex amplitudes in the agonist do not differ from the baseline, whereas those recorded in the uninvolved leg are larger. In other words: there is a differential effect.
3. After the RS the results for foot and finger movements are also different. With finger responses reflex amplitudes increase on both sides in a similar way. With foot movements a reversal of the differential effect takes place. Amplitudes in the involved leg increase with a steeper slope. Having reached a peak at about 4150 ms after the WS, they decrease below baseline. In the uninvolved leg they show a comparable picture to those with finger movements.

Since the bilateral increase in reflex amplitudes after the WS is present in all conditions, it is not selectively related to the preparatory process. As we mentioned already, the mere presentation of a tone also causes an increase. However, the signal value of the WS could also be of importance. Scheirs and Brunia (1982) have shown that besides an effect of the intensity of a tone there is an extra increase in reflex amplitudes due to the tone signaling the future arrival of an RS. This latter effect seems to be present later in time than that of the physical properties of the WS.

Reflex amplitudes are larger than the baseline in uninvolved muscles, both when a finger and when a foot response is prepared. This indicates that at the lumbar level an excitation of motor structures takes place both when the response to be given is produced at the cervical and at the lumbar level. Therefore, this excitation is part of an aselective preparatory process. A similar increase of the first component of the blink reflex has been found by Boelhouwer (1982) and Boelhouwer, Wijnen, and Brunia (1983). Thus, it could be suggested that this aselective excitation of motor structures during a foreperiod is a rather generalized phenomenon.

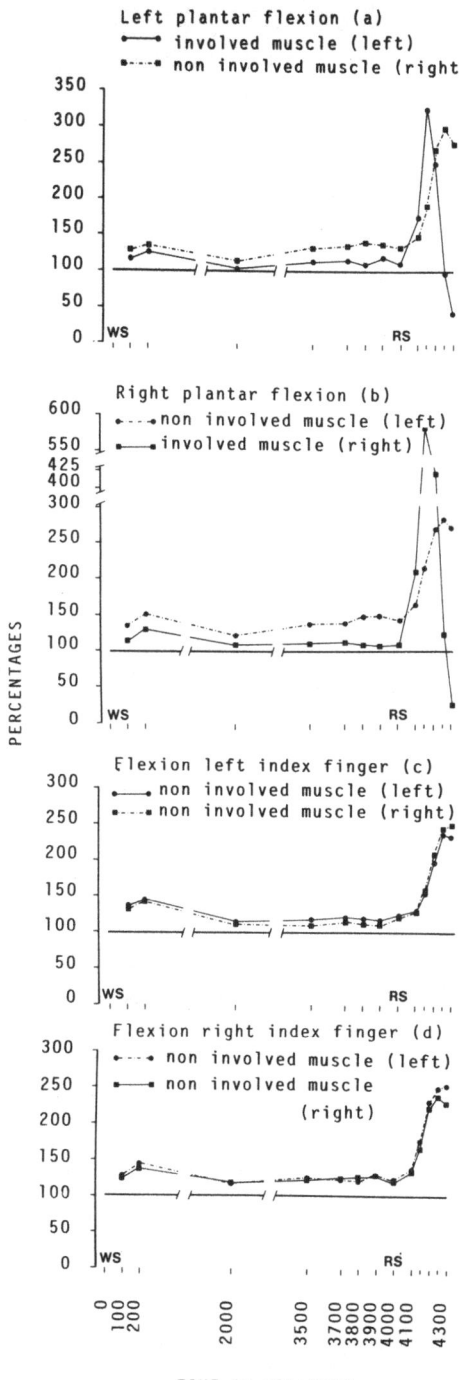

Fig. 17. Mean amplitudes of T reflexes evoked in both legs during and after a 4-s foreperiod of a simple RT experiment. Four response conditions: Condition A, left plantar flexion; Condition B, right plantar flexion; Condition C, left finger flexion; Condition D, right finger flexion. See also legend to Figure 14. (From Brunia, Scheirs, and Haagh 1982)

Reflex amplitudes in the agonist do not differ from the baseline. This selective preparatory sign seems to indicate that the motoneuron pool of the agonist is not facilitated. It has been shown, however, that prior to foot flexion movements human subjects sometimes tense their triceps surae muscles unintentionally and without the explicit instruction to do so (Burke, McKeon, Skuse and Westerman 1980; Haagh and Brunia 1984). When subjects were instructed to tense their triceps surae muscles voluntarily, T-reflex amplitudes were found to decrease even below baseline (Haagh, Spoeltman, Scheirs, and Brunia 1983). Thus it seems as if there is an agonist motoneuron output in such a situation, while the reflexes evoked via the same neurons are blocked. Requin, Bonnet, and Semjen (1977) postulated a presynaptic inhibitory influence acting on the Ia afferent fibers of the involved muscle to explain these results. In presynaptic inhibition, a mechanism which is widespread throughout the lower central nervous system, there is a depolarization of afferent fibers by axoaxonal synapses, causing a reduction of transmitter release at the afferent fiber terminal. Presynaptic inhibition of Ia afferents may be induced by volleys in afferent fibers from the homonymous muscle, from the ipsilateral flexor muscles, or by volleys in pathways from supraspinal centers (see Baldissera, Hultborn, and Illert 1981). The function of presynaptic inhibition in motor control, however, is not clear. Moreover, the mechanism seems to be rather generalized and not to be selective to one kind of muscle or to the muscles acting on one joint of a limb (Eccles 1964; McGeer, Eccles, and McGeer 1978). Therefore, some other explanations must be considered.

In the case of muscle contraction, for instance, there might be an increased muscle stiffness, which could reduce the effectiveness of the tendon tap in stretching the muscle. Another possibility is that during increased muscle tension there is occlusion of the reflex with motor units which are already active or which are in the refractory phase. This is an explanation proposed by Ott and Gassel (1969). And, finally, there is the possibility that the inhibition or lack of facilitation in the agonist muscle is caused by reciprocal inhibition from the antagonist, the tibialis anterior muscle. This third explanation is plausible, as Haagh and Brunia (1984) showed not only the EMG of the triceps surae muscle but also the EMG of the tibialis anterior muscle to be increased during the foreperiod. Evidence for Ia inhibitory actions from ankle flexors on extensors in subjects at rest was even provided by the fact that stimulation of the common peroneal nerve below or just above motor threshold was shown to inhibit the triceps surae Hoffmann reflex (Pierrot-Deseilligny, Morin, Bergego, and Tankov 1981; Shindo, Harayama, Kondo, Yanagisawa, and Tanaka 1984). The aselective excitation of motor structures during the foreperiod is likely to be due to descending influences from supraspinal origin. As no indication has been found for a selective activation of the fusimotor system in man, this reflex increase is probably due to a linked activation of alpha and gamma motor neurons or an activation of alpha motoneurons alone (Burke, Hagbarth, and Wallin 1980). The mechanism behind the lack of facilitation in the involved muscle, on the other hand, cannot as yet be established.

Following the RS, a transition from preparation to action takes place. Reflex amplitudes increase in all four conditions, pointing to the aselective aspect of this process. Agonists, however, also show a selective extra increase, which is steeper and reaches larger values, at least on the right side. The selective changes are related to the final command to execute the movement and to the execution itself. The aselective changes point to a supposedly generalized excitation of the motor system, which accompanies the execution of the movement.

In contrast to the first three experiments consistent changes in amplitude were found during the foreperiod in all four conditions. Preceding a finger flexion the pattern of changes was different from that preceding a plantar flexion of the foot. We interpret these two patterns as characteristic for motor preparation. Aselective aspects of the preparatory process are recorded prior to finger movements, and selective and aselective aspects prior to a plantar flexion of the foot. In the next experiment we will further investigate whether this interpretation is correct by comparing reflex changes prior to two different foot movements.

Reflex Changes Prior to Plantar Flexions and Dorsiflexions of the Foot

This experiment was aimed at the comparison of reflex changes prior to a plantar flexion and a dorsiflexion of the foot. Again four conditions were used. In Conditions A and B the response was a dorsiflexion on the right or left side, in Conditions C and D a plantar flexion.

Conditions C and D served as controls for the dorsiflexion. At the same time they functioned as a replication of the former experiment. The results of these conditions were comparable to the plantar flexion data of Fig. 17. Therefore only the results of Conditions A and B are shown here (see Fig. 18). The results can be summarized as follows:

1. After the WS a bilateral increase in amplitude is present, in all four conditions.
2. A differential effect is recorded during the remainder of the foreperiod prior to a plantar flexion of the foot. Preceding a dorsiflexion, reflex amplitudes are larger than the baseline on either side.
3. After the RS, amplitudes increase prior to a plantar flexion, whereas they decrease temporarily preceding a dorsiflexion.

As far as the influence of the WS is concerned, the results again point to an aselective increase in amplitude, since the kind of movement is irrelevant.

The differential effect prior to a plantar flexion on both sides has been replicated. It therefore underlines the interpretation given above. In line with our expectations, reflex amplitudes preceding a dorsiflexion were again larger than the baseline. This is in agreement with the results found prior to finger responses.

After the RS the picture is different for the two kinds of movements. With a plantar flexion the data are essentially the same as recorded in the former experiment. However, the reversal of the differential effect in the present experiment takes place 50 ms later. This suggests that the reversal of the differential effect is

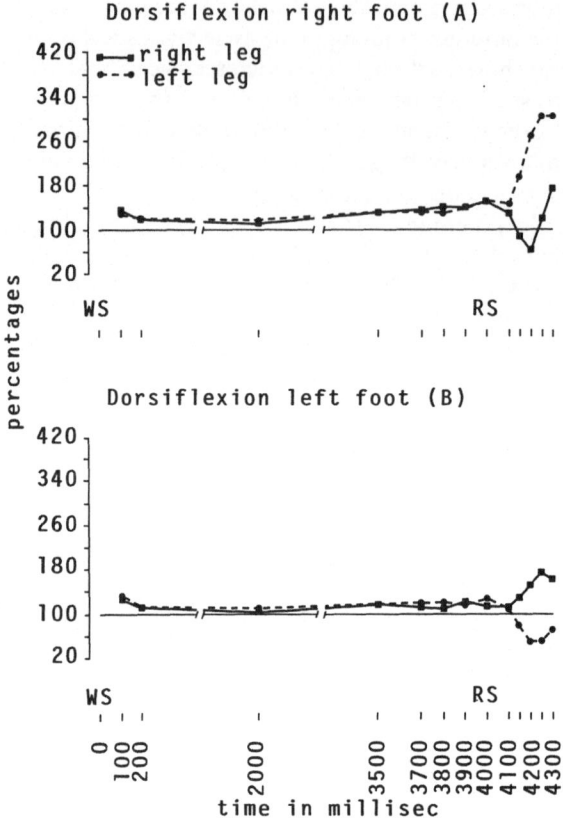

Fig. 18. Mean amplitudes of T reflexes evoked in both legs during and after a 4-s fore-period of a simple RT experiment. Responses were a dorsiflexion of the right foot (*A*) or a dorsiflexion of the left foot (*B*). See also legends to Figure 14. (From Brunia and Brocken, in preparation)

not time locked to the RS but to the movement. About 100 ms after the RS the amplitudes decrease prior to a dorsiflexion. This is presumably the consequence of the reciprocal innervation of the motoneurons of the tibialis anterior muscle and the soleus muscle. In other words, the soleus functions as antagonist only after the presentation of the RS, presumably at the onset of the dorsiflexion.

So far the results are rather consistent. A differential effect is present prior to a plantar flexion of the foot and not prior to a finger flexion or a dorsiflexion of the foot. The differential effect is composed of an aselective and a selective process. The aselective changes were defined as not related to the agonist. They seem to represent a more general process at the lumbosacral level, but perhaps the whole neuraxis, prior to different movements. This activation of the motor system, which is possibly largely subliminal, might be related to the maintenance of posture as a prerequisite for a foot response. On the other hand, the selective aspect might be related to the defense of the agonist motoneuron pool against disturbing influences from the periphery, its function being to keep the motoneurons ready for the final command (Requin et al. 1977).

We have found a consistent pattern of changes in reflex amplitudes preceding a plantar flexion of the foot. We consider the differential effect during the foreperiod as a specific aspect of motor preparation. Another way of testing this is creating conditions in which response probability is systematically manipulated. Therefore a Go–No Go experiment was done.

Reflex Changes as a Function of Response Probability

T reflexes were evoked bilaterally during the foreperiod and shortly after the RS in three conditions with different response probabilities: .80, .50, and .20 (Conditions A, B, and C, respectively). The results are summarized in Fig. 19. Since subjects had to react in most of the trials of Condition A, motor preparation was expected to be strongest here. In line with this hypothesis a differential effect was present indeed in this and not in the other two conditions. In the latter conditions reflex amplitudes were not significantly different between legs, and at most of the points in time they were larger than the baseline. Thus the selective aspects of preparation were only found when motor preparation was high. In both other conditions the aselective aspects showed up again as an increase in reflex amplitudes above baseline.

Summarizing our reflex data, we have found the following results:

1. T-reflex amplitudes are not systematically different from the baseline if no response is prepared.
2. T-reflex amplitudes are systematically larger than the baseline if evoked in muscles uninvolved in the prepared response.
3. T-reflex amplitudes in involved muscles are systematically smaller than those evoked in muscles uninvolved in the response.
4. This differential effect is only present with a high response probability.

In the final pages of this chapter we will turn to the question of a possible relationship between the results of the reflex experiments and those of the slow potential studies.

The Cortical and Spinal Level

The major question in comparing the psychophysiological changes at the cortical and at the spinal level is whether the spinal changes are cortically controlled during the total length of a foreperiod or whether they are relatively independent of cortical processes. In the first case one might expect a parallelism between the cortical and peripheral measures of motor preparation. We will discuss the suc-

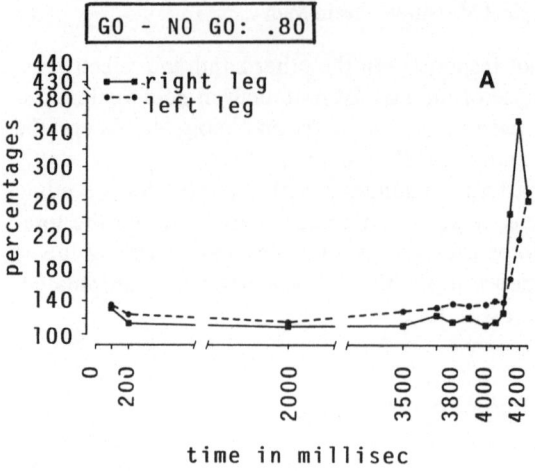

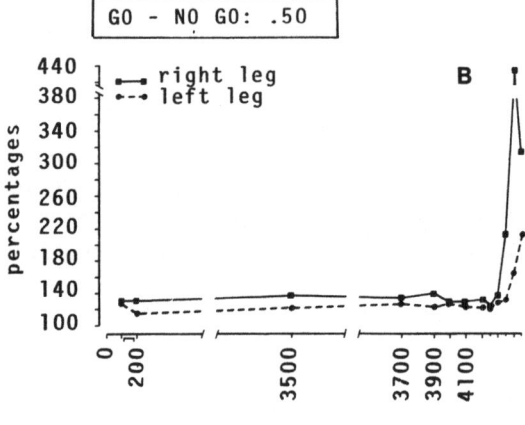

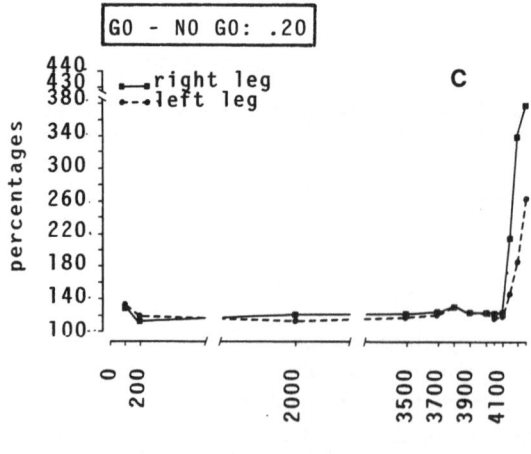

Fig. 19 A–C. Mean amplitudes of T reflexes evoked in both legs during and after a 4-s foreperiod of a Go–No Go experiment. Three different response probabilities: $p = .80$, $p = .50$, and $p = .20$. Responses were a plantar flexion of the right foot. See also legends to Figure 14

cessive cortical phenomena, recorded from the presentation of the WS until the movement, and see whether spinal processes may or may not be related to them.

The first electrophysiological phenomenon which can be recorded at the cortical level during the foreperiod of a RT experiment is the event-related potential (ERP) following the WS. At about the same time an increase in reflex amplitude is found at the spinal level. It is known that the early so-called exogenous components of the ERP (< 100 ms) reflect the physical properties of the stimulus (Donchin, Ritter, and McCallum 1978). The same seems to hold for the increase in reflex amplitudes, at least after an auditory stimulus. Scheirs and Brunia (1982) found such an increase after a loud but not after a soft tone, in agreement with earlier results of Davis and Beaton (1968). This points to a disinhibition or facilitation of the motoneurons in question related to the physical aspects of the stimulus. As soon as the same tone serves as a WS in an RT experiment, the reflex amplitudes remain elevated over a longer period. This sustained excitability increase of spinal motorstructures coincides with the first endogenous ERP components. First, a processing negativity occurs which has a very short latency (50–150 ms) and is associated with orienting to, and further processing of, a relevant stimulus (Näätänen and Michie, 1979). The negativity overlaps the N100 component and may continue for 500 ms. The P300 reflects the termination of these stimulus evaluation processes (Duncan-Johnson and Donchin 1977). We assume that, at this very moment, preparatory processes are started. It is important to note that the cortical processes of stimulus detection, evaluation, and decision are concomitant with an aselective increased excitability of the spinal motorstructures.

Following the ERP the early CNV wave is the next cortical phenomenon. It reaches its maximum at about 750 ms after the WS (see Fig. 6) and reflects processes in the frontal lobe which are related to orienting. Orienting implies not only a turning to the stimulus, but also a number of physiological changes aimed at a future action (Lynn 1966). Although we have no reflex data available at about 750 ms after the WS, we found enlarged amplitudes at both 500 and 1000 ms (Scheirs and Brunia, in press). We note that this indication of an increased excitability of the motoneurons coincides with the frontal negativity and that it, therefore, might be related to the orienting response. Considering the reflex literature, we assume that the increased reflex amplitudes during this epoch are related to aselective preparation.

Preparation for a movement in a situation which allows the subject to plan and time the movement goes along with a slow negative shift which begins about 1.5 s prior to that movement. The sources of that activity are found in the premotor and motor cortex and might also be present in the supplementary motor area. It has been suggested that the premotor cortex is more related to the planning of the movement and the motor cortex to its execution. Planning seems to be an affair for both hemispheres, execution for the hemisphere contralateral to the movement side. We would like to point out the fact that the negative shift is present over the motor cortex of both hemispheres. This indicates that both motor cortices are active during the preparation, the hemisphere differences in RP amplitude pointing to the privileged role of the contralateral motor cortex. Should there be a coherence between the cortical and spinal measures of preparation, one would expect the bilateral RP to be related to aselective spinal changes and the hemisphere differences to the differential effect. Further research will be necessary to evaluate these hypotheses, but we expect much more complicated relations. It has been shown, for example, that spinal and cortical measures can be influenced by instructed muscle tension in a different way. If subjects are taught to tense their calf muscles during the foreperiod in order to reach shorter RTs, the differential effect in reflex amplitudes is found to be larger than when the calf muscles are relaxed (Haagh, Spoeltman, Scheirs and Brunia 1983). In this case a clear relation between performance, surface EMG, and reflex changes . was found.

In a similar experiment Gaillard et al. (1980) compared CNV late wave amplitudes under instructed tension and relaxation of the agonist. The late wave was not attenuated in the relaxed as compared with the tensed condition. Contrary to this dissociation between EMG and EEG measures of preparation, a parallelism between these measures was found by Brunia and Vingerhoets (1980). These authors reported larger CNV late waves preceding fast than preceding slow responses (see Fig. 6). Parallel to these changes the slight surface EMG activity in the agonist was more pronounced prior to fast than to slow movements. In other words, the instruction in the experiment of Gaillard et al. (1980) caused another organization of the preparatory processes than was found in the spontaneous behavior of the subjects in the study of Brunia and Vingerhoets (1980). Whether or not a parallelism shows up is dependent on the subject's response strategy. If the subjects are free to choose, they may indeed try to stay as close as possible to the motor action limit by a depolarization of the agonist motoneurons without reaching their firing threshold. Since this is difficult to achieve, some of the motoneurons might fire, resulting in a slight EMG activity but not in movement. Presumably, that is what Brunia and Vingerhoets (1980) have found.

Following the RP, the MP or N_2 is the next electrophysiological phenomenon recorded prior to the movement. This increase in negativity reflects the firing of the pyramidal tract neurons, which will cause the final depolarization of the alpha motoneurons in the spinal cord. The reflex data suggest that the reversal of the differential effect, if present, and the sharp increase in reflex amplitude in the agonist after the RS indicate the arrival of the excitatory impulses on the motoneurons, which results in the movement. This suggestion was corroborated by EMG data (Haagh et al. 1983).

A simplified picture of the neuronal structures possibly involved in information processing and movement execution during a warned RT experiment is given in Fig. 20. Presentation of a tone results in activation of area 22, after crossing a number of brain stem synapses in the auditory pathways. The first large peak of the auditory ERP is the N 100, originating presumably from area 22 or its surroundings (Vaughan and Ritter 1970). One hundred milliseconds is sufficient for it to pass a brain stem-cortex-spinal cord loop. However, since the early facilitation of the motoneurons in the spinal cord coincides with the peak of the N 100

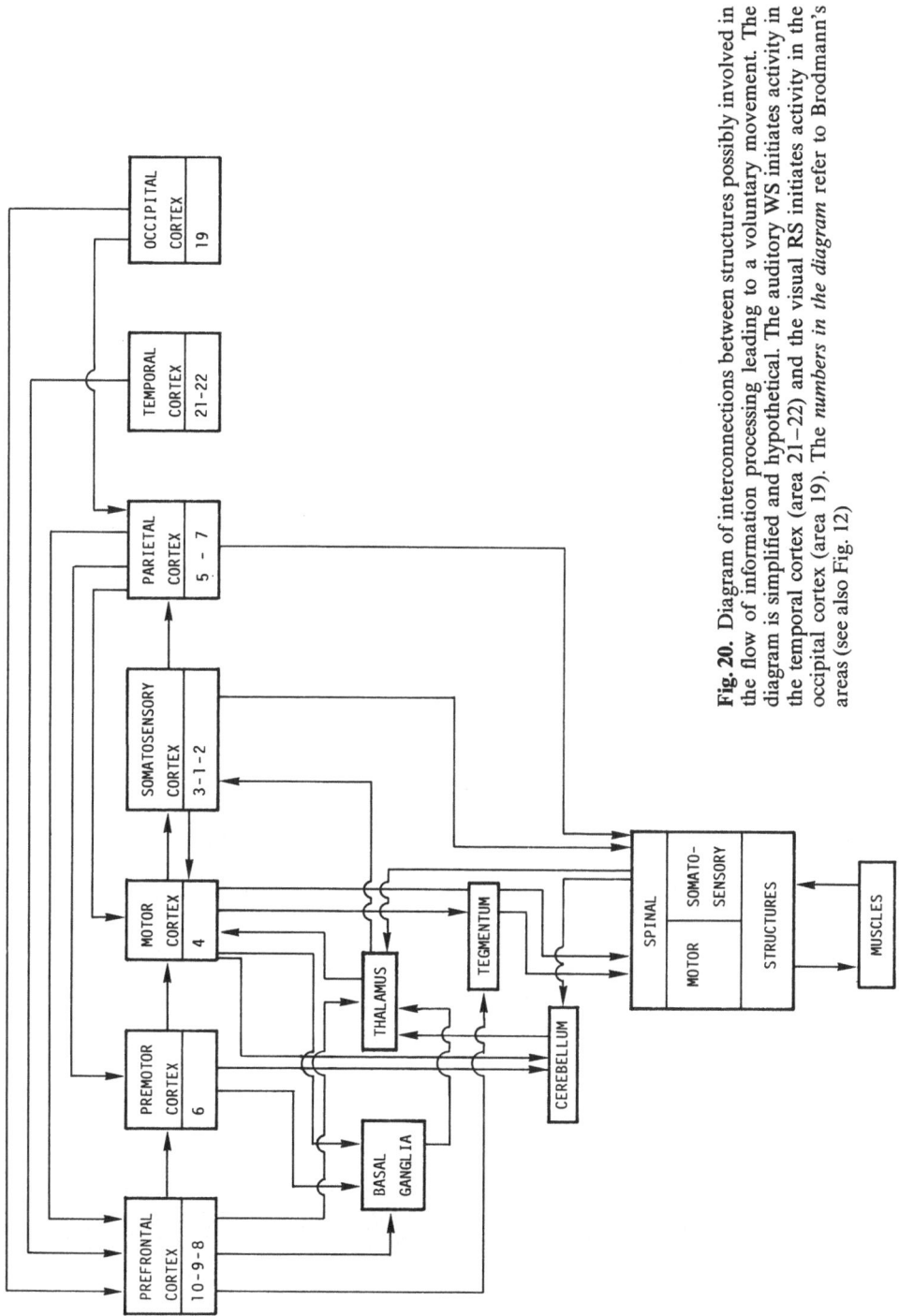

Fig. 20. Diagram of interconnections between structures possibly involved in the flow of information processing leading to a voluntary movement. The diagram is simplified and hypothetical. The auditory WS initiates activity in the temporal cortex (area 21–22) and the visual RS initiates activity in the occipital cortex (area 19). The *numbers in the diagram* refer to Brodmann's areas (see also Fig. 12)

component we think this to be an argument for an auditory subcorticospinal facilitation, in which the reticular formation might play a role. The pathway, possibly indirect, from area 22 to the prefrontal cortex (Jones and Powell 1970) might be the way via which the latter becomes activated. The end of the evaluation of the significance of the WS is marked by the P300 component, which is maximal at the vertex. As was indicated earlier, this does not imply that the source of this component is localized in the parietal cortex (Wood, Allison, Goff, Williamson, and Spencer 1980). It is not known whether the onset of the activation of the prefrontal cortex starts before or after the emergence of the P300, although the surface EEG recordings show the slow wave after the P300. The prefrontal cortex is related to orienting and possibly also to mnemonic processes. Since ERP components earlier than 300 ms have been found, which are related to orienting (Näätänen 1982), this could be an argument to suppose that the prefrontal cortex is brought into action before the P300 becomes manifest.

The premotor cortex is the next brain structure to be activated, its function – among others – being the timing of the response. It is accompanied by the RP. Important subcortical structures as, e.g., basal ganglia and cerebellum, receive the major output from the premotor cortex. This might be of importance for the programming of the movement together with the setting of postural adjustments, necessary to create a starting point for the movement. At the cortical level this is almost immediately followed by an activation of the motor cortex. As a consequence an RP is also recorded here. At the spinal level this might result in a generalized increase in the excitability of motoneurons, reflected by the increased T-reflex amplitudes. The presentation of the RS, which in our experiments was a visual stimulus, arrives at area 17 and is processed in areas 18 and 19. The latter is known to activate area 7 of the parietal cortex (Wiesendanger 1981) via which the premotor cortex can be reached again. The ERP following the RS coincides in time with the PMP, which is supposed to be the command to move (Deecke and Kornhuber 1977). Basal ganglia and cerebellum are possibly the intermediate stations before, via the thalamus, the motor cortex is activated. From there the final command is transmitted to the spinal motoneurons of the agonist. The electrophysiological reflection of this is the motor potential (N2), which is followed by the reversal of the differential effect found with T reflexes and the sharp increase in amplitude of the T reflexes evoked in the agonist.

The recording of EEG and EMG during the foreperiod of RT experiments in man has of course its disadvantages. Very complicated processes both within the cortex and subcortical centra, and interaction between different levels of the CNS, remain inaccessible for this recording technique. Recording of MUA and slow potentials in animals, especially in monkeys, can help us further in understanding the origin of psychophysiological data obtained in man. However, the brain of *Homo sapiens* is much more complicated than that of a monkey. In spite of this difficulty, our work is aimed at the understanding of what is going on in the human brain. On epistemiological and ethical grounds this task is comparable to trying to reach the horizon.

References

Arezzo, J., and Vaughan, Jr., H. G. (1975). Cortical potentials associated with voluntary movements in the monkey. Brain Research, 88, 99–104.

Arezzo, J., and Vaughan, Jr., H. G. (1980). Cortical sources and surface topography of the motor potential and somatosensory evoked potential in the monkey. In H. H. Kornhuber and L. Deecke (Eds.), Motivation, motor and sensory processes of the brain: Electrical potentials, behavior and clinical use. Progress in brain research, Vol. 54 (pp. 77––83). Amsterdam: Elsevier.

Arezzo, J., Vaughan, Jr., H. G., and Koss, B. (1977). Relationship of neuronal activity to gross movement-related potentials in monkey pre- and postcentral cortex. Brain Research, 132, 362–369.

Baldissera, F., Hultborn, H., and Illert, M. (1981). Integration in spinal neuronal systems. In J. M. Brookhart and V. B. Mountcastle (Eds.), Handbook of physiology, the nervous system, Vol. II, part 1 (pp. 509–596). Bethesda: American Physiological Society.

Beale, D. K. (1971). Facilitation of the knee jerk as a function of the interval between auditory and stretching stimuli. Psychophysiology, 8, 504–508.

Biedenbach, M. A., and Stevens, C. F. (1969). Electrical activity in cat olfactory cortex produced by synchronous orthodromic volleys. Journal of Neurophysiology, 32, 193–203.

Boelhouwer, A. J. W. (1982). Blink reflexes and preparation. Biological Psychology, 14, 277–285.

Boelhouwer, A. J. W., Wijnen, J. L. C., and Brunia, C. H. M. (1983). Changes of human blink reflex magnitude during a fixed foreperiod of 3 sec. The International Journal of Neuroscience, 18, 231–238.

Borda, R. P. (1970). The effect of altered drive states on the contingent negative variation (CNV) in Rhesus Monkeys. Electroencephalography and Clinical Neurophysiology, 29, 173–180.

Brunia, C. H. M. (1984). Selective and aselective control of spinal motor structures during preparation for a movement. In: S. Kornblum and J. Requin (Eds.), Preparatory states and processes (pp. 285–302). Hillsdale: Erlbaum

Brunia, C. H. M., and Van den Bosch, W. E. J. (1984). The influence of response side on the readiness potential prior to finger and foot movements (a preliminary report). In R. Karrer, J. Cohen, and P. Tueting (Eds.), Brain and information: Event related potentials (pp. 434–437). New York: Academic Sciences.

Brunia, C. H. M., and Vingerhoets, A. J. J. M. (1980). CNV and EMG preceding a plantar flexion of the foot. Biological Psychology, 11, 181–191.

Brunia, C. H. M., and Vingerhoets, A. J. J. M. (1981). Opposite hemisphere differences in movement related potentials preceding foot and finger flexion. Biological Psychology, 13, 261–269.

Brunia, C. H. M., Scheirs, J. G. M., and Haagh, S. A. V. M. (1982). Changes of Achilles tendon reflexes during a fixed foreperiod of four seconds. Psychophysiology, 19, 63–70.

Burke, D., Hagbarth, K. E., and Wallin, B. G. (1980). Alpha-gamma linkage and the mechanisms of reflex reinforcement. In J. E. Desmedt (Ed.), Spinal and supraspinal mechanisms of voluntary motor control and locomotion. Progress in clinical neurophysiology, Vol. 8 (pp. 170–180). Basel: Karger.

Burke, D., McKeon, B., Skuse, N. F., and Westerman, R. A. (1980). Anticipation and fusimotor activity in preparation for a voluntary contraction. Journal of Physiology, 306, 337–348.

Callaway, E. (1975). Brain electrical potentials and individual differences. New York: Grune and Stratton.

Caspers, H., Speckmann, E. J., and Lehmenkühler, A. (1980). Electrogenesis of cortical DC potentials. In H. H. Kornhuber and L. Deecke (Eds.), Motivation, motor and sensory processes of the brain: Electrical potentials, behavior and clinical use. Progress in brain research, Vol. 54 (pp. 3–15). Amsterdam: Elsevier.

Cohen, J. (1969). Very slow brain potentials relating to expectancy: The CNV. In E. Donchin and D. B. Lindsley (Eds.), Average evoked potentials (pp. 143–198). Washington D.C.: NASA SP-191.

Connor, W. H., and Lang, P. J. (1969). Cortical slow-wave and cardiac rate response in stimulus orientation and reaction time conditions. Journal of Experimental Psychology, 82, 310–320.

Davis, C. M., and Beaton, R. D. (1968). Facilitation and adaptation of the human quadriceps stretch reflex produced by auditory stimulation. Journal of Comparative and Physiological Psychology, 66, 483–487.

Deecke, L., and Kornhuber, H. H. (1977). Cerebral potentials and the initiation of voluntary movement. In J. E. Desmedt (Ed.), Attention, voluntary contraction and event-related cerebral potentials. Progress in clinical neurophysiology, Vol. 1 (pp. 132–150). Basel: Karger.

Deecke, L., Becker, W., Grözinger, B., and Kriebel, J. (1976). CNV-Bereitschaftspotential relationships. In W. C. McCallum and J. R. Knott (Eds.), The responsive brain (pp. 214–216). Bristol: Wright.

Donchin, E., Otto, D., Gerbrandt, L. K., and Pribram, K. H. (1971). While a monkey waits: Electrocortical events recorded during the foreperiod of a reaction time study. Electroencephalography and Clinical Neurophysiology, 31, 115–127.

Donchin, E., Gerbrandt, L. A., Leifer, L., and Tucker, L. (1972). Is the contingent negative variation contingent on a motor response? Psychophysiology, 9, 178–188.

Donchin, E., Callaway, E., Cooper, R., Desmedt, J. E., Goff, W. R., Hillyard, S. A., and Sutton, S. (1977). Publication criteria for studies of evoked potentials (EP) in man. In J. E. Desmedt (Ed.), Attention, voluntary contraction and event related cerebral potentials. Progress in clinical neurophysiology, Vol. 1 (pp. 1–11). Basel: Karger.

Donchin, E., Kutas, M., and McCarthy, G. (1977). Electrocortical indices of hemispheric utilization. In R. W. Doty, L. Goldstein, J. Jaynes, and G. Kranthamer (Eds.), Lateralization in the nervous system (pp. 339–384). New York: Academic Press.

Donchin, E., Ritter, W., and McCallum, W. C. (1978). Cognitive psychophysiology: the endogenous components of the ERP. In E. Callaway, P. Tueting, and S. H. Koslow (Eds.), Event related brain potentials in man (pp. 349–411). New York: Academic Press.

Duncan-Johnson, C. C. and Donchin, E. (1977). On quantifying surprise: the variation of event-related potentials with subjective probability. Psychophysiology, 14, 456–467.

Eccles, J. C. (1964). Presynaptic inhibition in the spinal cord. In J. C. Eccles, and J. P. Schadé (Eds.), Physiology of spinal neurons. Progress in brain research, Vol. 12 (pp. 65–91). Amsterdam: Elsevier.

Evarts, E. V. (1981). Role of motor cortex in voluntary movements in primates. In J. M. Brookhart and V. B. Mountcastle (Eds.), The nervous system, Handbook of physiology, Vol. II, part 2 (pp. 1083–1120). Bethesda: American Physiological Society.

Fuster, J. M. (1981). Prefrontal cortex in motor control. In J. M. Brookhart and V. B. Mountcastle (Eds.), Handbook of physiology, The nervous system, Vol. II, part 2 (pp. 1149–1178). Bethesda: American Physiological Society.

Fuster, J. M., and Alexander, G. E. (1971). Neuron activity related to short term memory. Science, 173, 652–654.

Gaillard, A. W. K. (1976). Effects of warning-signal modality on the contingent negative variation (CNV). Biological Psychology, 4, 139–154.

Gaillard, A. W. K. (1980). Cortical correlates of motor preparation. In R. S. Nickerson (Ed.), Attention and performance VIII (pp. 75–91). Hillsdale: Erlbaum.

Gaillard, A. W. K., Perdok, J., and Varey, C. A. (1980). Motor preparation at a cortical and at a peripheral level. In H. H. Kornhuber and L. Deecke (Eds.), Motivation, motor and sensory processes of the brain: electrical potentials, behavior and clinical use. Progress in brain research, Vol. 54 (pp. 214–218). Amsterdam: Elsevier.

Gemba, H., Hashimoto, S., and Sasaki, K. (1979). Slow potentials preceding self paced hand movements in the parietal cortex of monkeys. Neuroscience Letters, 15, 87–92.

Gemba, H., Sasaki, K., and Hashimoto, S. (1980). Distribution of premovement slow cortical potentials associated with self-paced hand movements in monkeys. Neuroscience Letters, 20, 159–163.

Gerbrandt, L. K. (1977). Analysis of movement potential components. In J. E. Desmedt (Ed.), Attention, voluntary contraction and event-related cerebral potentials. Progress in clinical neurophysiology, Vol. 1 (pp. 174–188). Basel: Karger.

Gerbrandt, L. K., Goff, W. R., and Smith, D. B. (1973). Distribution of the human average movement potential. Electroencephalography and Clinical Neurophysiology, 34, 461–474.

Gilden, L., Vaughan, Jr., H. G., and Costa, L. D. (1966). Summated human EEG potentials with voluntary movement. Electroencephalography and Clinical Neurophysiology, 20, 433–438.

Gross, C. G., and Weiskrantz, L. (1964). Some changes in behavior produced by lateral frontal lesions in the Macaque. In J. M. Warren, and K. Akert (Eds.), The frontal granular cortex and behavior (pp. 74–101). New York: McGraw Hill.

Haagh, S. A. V. M., and Brunia, C. H. M. (1984). Cardiac-somatic coupling during the foreperiod in a simple reaction time task. Psychological Research, 46, 3–13.

Haagh, S. A. V. M., and Brunia, C. H. M. (1985). Anticipatory response-relevant muscle activity, CNV amplitude and simple reaction time. Electroencephalography and Clinical Neurophysiology, in press.

Haagh, S. A. V. M., Spoeltman, W. T. E., Scheirs, J. G. M., and Brunia, C. H. M. (1983). Surface EMG and Achilles tendon reflex amplitudes during a foot movement in a reaction time task. Biological Psychology, 17, 81–96.

Hablitz, J. J. (1973). Operant conditioning and slow potential changes from monkey cortex. Electroencephalography and Clinical Neurophysiology, 34, 399–408.

Hashimoto, S., Gemba, H., and Sasaki, K. (1979). Analysis of slow cortical potentials preceding self-paced hand movements in the monkey. Experimental Neurology, 65, 218–229.

Hashimoto, S., Gemba, H., and Sasaki, K. (1980). Premovement slow cortical potentials and required muscle force in self-paced hand movements in the monkey. Brain Research, 197, 415–423.

Hillard, S. A. (1973). The CNV and human behavior. In W. C. McCallum and J. R. Knott (Eds.), Event-related slow potentials of the brain. Their relations to behavior. Electroencephalography and Clinical Neurophysiology [Suppl.], 3, 161–171.

Hillyard, S. A., and Galambos, R. (1967). Effects of stimulus and response contingencies on a surface negative slow potential shift in man. Electroencephalography and Clinical Neurophysiology, 22, 297–304.

Hyvarinen, J., and Poranen, A. (1974). Function of the parietal associative area 7 as revealed from cellular discharges in alert monkeys. Brain, 97, 673–692.

Irwin, D. A., Knott, J. R., McAdam, D. W., and Rebert, C. S. (1966). Motivational determinants of the "contingent negative variation". Electroencephalography and Clinical Neurophysiology, 21, 538–543.

Järvilehto, T., and Frühstorfer, H. (1970). Differentiations between slow cortical potentials associated with motor and mental acts in man. Experimental Brain Research, 11, 309–317.

Jones, E. G., and Powell, T. P. S. (1970). An anatomical study of converging sensory pathways within the cerebral cortex of the monkey. Brain, 93, 793–820.

Knott, J. R., and Irwin, D. A. (1973). Anxiety, stress and the contingent negative variation. Archives of General Psychiatry, 29, 538–541.

Klorman, R., and Bentsen, E. (1975). Effects of warning signal duration on the early and late components of the contingent negative variation. Biological Psychology, 3, 263–275.

Kornhuber, H. H. (1974). Cerebral cortex, cerebellum and basal ganglia: an introduction to their motor functions. In F. O. Schmitt, and F. G. Worden (Eds.), The neurosciences, Third Study Program (pp. 276–280). Cambridge, MIT Press.

Kornhuber, H. H., and Deecke, L. (1965). Hirnpotentialänderungen bei Willkür-bewegungen und passiven Bewegungen des Menschen: Bereitschaftspotential und re-afferente Potentiale. Pflügers Archiv, *284*, 1–17.

Kutas, M., and Donchin, E. (1977). The effect of handedness, of responding hand and of response force on the contralateral dominance of the readiness potential. In J. E. Desmedt (Ed.), Attention, voluntary contraction and event-related cerebral potentials. Progress in Clinical Neurophysiology, Vol. 1 (pp. 189–210). Basel: Karger.

Lacey, J. I., and Lacey, B. C. (1970). Some autonomic-central nervous system interrelationships. In P. Black (Ed.), Physiological correlates of emotion (pp. 205–228). New York: Academic.

Lamarre, Y., Spidalieri, G., Burby, L., and Lund, J. P. (1980). Programming of initiation and execution of ballistic arm movements in the monkey. In H. H. Kornhuber and L. Deecke (Eds.), Motivation, motor and sensory processes of the brain: electrical potentials, behavior and clinical use. Progress in brain research, Vol. 54 (pp. 157–169). Amsterdam: Elsevier.

Lang, P. J., Öhman, A., and Simons, R. F. (1978). The psychophysiology of anticipation. In J. Requin (Ed.), Attention and performance VII (pp. 460–485). Hillsdale: Erlbaum.

Libet, B., Wright, Jr., E. W., and Gleason, C. A. (1982). Readiness potentials preceding unrestricted 'spontaneous' vs. preplanned voluntary acts. Electroencephalography and Clinical Neurophysiology, *54*, 322–335.

Loveless, N. E. (1975). The effect of warning interval on signal detection and event-related slow potentials in the brain. Perception and Psychophysics, *17*, 565–570.

Loveless, N. E. (1976). Distribution of responses to non signal stimuli. In W. C. McCallum, and J. R. Knott (Eds.), The responsive brain (pp. 26–29). Bristol: Wright.

Loveless, N. E. (1979). Event related slow potentials of the brain as expressions of orienting functions. In H. D. Kimmel, E. H. van Olst, and J. F. Orlebeke (Eds.), The orienting reflex in humans (pp. 77–100). Hillsdale: Erlbaum.

Loveless, N. E., and Sanford, A. J. (1974a). Effects of age on the contingent negative variation and preparatory set in a reaction-time task. Journal of Gerontology, *29*, 52–63.

Loveless, N. E., and Sanford, A. J. (1974b). Slow potential correlates of preparatory set. Biological Psychology, *1*, 303–314.

Loveless, N. E., and Sanford, A. J. (1975). The impact of warning signal intensity on reaction time and components of the contingent negative variation. Biological Psychology, *2*, 217–226.

Low, M. D., and McSherry, J. W. (1968). Further observations of psychological factors involved in CNV genesis. Electroencephalography and Clinical Neurophysiology, *25*, 203–207.

Low, M. D., Borda, R. P., Frost, J. D., and Kellaway, P. (1966). Surface negative slow potential shift associated with conditioning in man. Neurology (Minneap.), *16*, 711–782.

Luria, A. R., and Homskaya, E. D. (1970). Frontal lobes and the regulation of arousal processes. In D. T. Mostofsky (Ed.), Attention: contemporary theory and analysis (pp. 303–330). New York: Appleton-Century-Crofts.

Lynn, R. (1966). Attention, arousal and the orientation reaction. Oxford: Pergamon.

McAdam, D. W. (1974). The contingent negative variations. In R. F. Thompson and M. M. Patterson (Eds.), Bioelectric recording techniques, part B (pp. 245–257). New York: Academic Press.

McAdam, D. W., Knott, J. R., and Rebert, C. S. (1969). Cortical slow potential changes in man related to interstimulus interval. Psychophysiology, *5*, 349–358.

McCallum, W. C. (1978). Relationships between Bereitschaftspotential and contingent negative variation. In D. A. Otto (Ed.), Multidisciplinary perspectives in event-related potential research (pp. 124–130). Washington: U.S. Government Printing Office.

McCallum, W. C., and Walter, W. G. (1968). The effects of attention and distraction on the contingent negative variation in normal and neurotic subjects. Electroencephalography and Clinical Neurophysiology, *25*, 319–329.

McCallum, W. C., Papakostopoulos, D., Gombi, R., Winter, A. L., Cooper, R., and Griffith, H. B. (1973. Event related slow potential changes in human brain stem. Nature, *242*, 465–467.

McGeer, P. L., Eccles, J. C., and McGeer, E. G. (1978). Molecular neurobiology of the mammalian brain (pp. 135–138). New York: Plenum.

McSherry, J. W., Borda, R. P., and Hablitz, J. J. (1977). Analysis of event related slow potentials in primates. In J. E. Desmedt (Ed.), Attention, voluntary contraction and event-related cerebral potentials. Progress in clinical neurophysiology, Vol. 1 (pp. 231–243). Basel: Karger.

Milner, B. (1974). Hemispheric specialisation: scope and limits. In F. O. Schmidt, and F. G. Worden (Eds.), The neurosciences, Third study program (pp. 75–89). Cambridge: MIT Press.

Näätänen, R. (1982). Processing negativity: an evoked-potential reflection of selective attention. Psychological Bulletin, *92*, 605–640.

Näätänen, R., and Michie, P. T. (1979). Early selective attention effects on the evoked potential: a critical review and reinterpretation. Biological Psychology, *8*, 81–136.

Niemi, P., and Näätänen, R. (1981). Foreperiod and simple reaction time. Psychological Bulletin, *89*, 133–162.

Ott, K. H., and Gassel, M. M. (1969). Methods of tendon jerk reinforcement. The role of muscle activity in reflex excitability. Journal of Neurology, Neurosurgery and Psychiatry, *32*, 541–547.

Paillard, J. (1955). Réflexes et régulations d'origine proprioceptive chez l'homme. Paris: Librairie Arnette.

Perdok, J., and Gaillard, A. W. K. (1979). The terminal CNV and stimulus discriminability in motor and sensory tasks. Biological Psychology, *8*, 213–223.

Pierrot-Deseilligny, E., Morin, C., Bergego, C., and Tankov, N. (1981). Pattern of group I fibre projections from ankle flexor and extensor muscles in man. Experimental Brain Research, *42*, 337–350.

Rebert, C. S. (1972). Cortical and subcortical slow potentials in the monkey's brain during a preparatory interval. Electroencephalography and Clinical Neurophysiology, *23*, 389–402.

Rebert, C. S. (1973). Slow potential correlates of neuronal population responses in the cat's lateral geniculate nucleus. Electroencephalography and Clinical Neurophysiology, *35*, 511–515.

Rebert, C. S. (1977). Intracerebral slow potential changes in monkeys during the foreperiod of reaction time. In J. E. Desmedt (Ed.), Attention, voluntary contraction and event-related cerebral potentials. Progress in clinical neurophysiology, Vol. I (pp. 242–253). Basel: Karger.

Rebert, C. S., McAdam, D. W., Knott, J. R., and Irwin, D. A. (1976). Slow potential changes in human related to level of motivation. Journal of Comparative Physiological Psychology, *63*, 20–33.

Requin, J., Bonnet, M., and Semjen, A. (1977). Is there a specificity in the supraspinal control of motor structures during preparation? In S. Dornic (Ed.), Attention and performance VI (pp. 139–174). Hillsdale: Erlbaum.

Rohrbaugh, J. W., and Gaillard, A. W. K. (1983). Sensory and motor aspects of the contingent negative variation. In A. W. K. Gaillard and W. Ritter (Eds.), Tutorials in ERP research: Endogenous components (pp. 269–311). Amsterdam: North-Holland.

Rohrbaugh, J. W., Syndulko, K., and Lindsley, D. B. (1976). Brain wave components of the contingent negative variation in humans. Science, *191*, 1055–1057.

Rossignol, S., and Melvill-Jones, G. (1976). Audio-spinal influence in man studied by the H reflex and its possible role on rhythmic movements synchronized to sound. Electroencephalography and Clinical Neurophysiology, *41*, 83–92.

Scheirs, J. G. M., and Brunia, C. H. M. (1982). Effects of stimulus and task factors on Achilles Tendon reflexes evoked early during a preparatory period. Physiology and Behavior, *28*, 681–685.

Scheirs, J. G. M., and Brunia, C. H. M. (1985). Achilles Tendon reflexes and surface EMG activity during anticipation of a significant event and preparation for a voluntary movement. Journal of Motor Behavior, in press.

Shibasaki, H., Barret, G., Halliday, E., and Halliday, A. M. (1980). Components of the movement-related cortical potential and their scalp topography. Electroencephalography and Clinical Neurophysiology, 49, 213–226.

Shibasaki, H., Barret, G., Halliday, E., and Halliday, A. M. (1981). Cortical potentials associated with voluntary foot movement in man. Electroencephalography and Clinical Neurophysiology, 52, 507–516.

Shindo, M., Harayama, H., Kondo, U., Yanagisawa, N., and Tanaka, R. (1984). Changes in reciprocal I a inhibition during voluntary contractions in man. Experimental Brain Research, 53, 400–408.

Stamm, J. S., and Rosen, S. C. (1973). The locus and crucial time of implication of prefrontal cortex in the delayed response task. In K. H. Pribram and A. R. Luria (Eds.), Psychophysiology of the frontal lobes (pp. 139–153). New York: Academic Press.

Tanji, J., Taniguchi, K., and Saga, T. (1980). Supplementary motor area: neuronal response to motor instruction. Journal of Neurophysiology, 43, 1, 60–68.

Tecce, T. J. (1972). Contingent negative variation (CNV) and psychological processes in man. Psychological Bulletin, 77, 73–108.

Tecce, J. J., and Cattanach, L. (1982). Contingent negative variation. In E. Niedermeyer and F. Lopez da Silva (Eds.), Electroencephalography (pp. 543–562. Baltimore: Urban and Schwarzenberg.

Vaughan, H. G. Jr., and Ritter, W. (1970). The sources of auditory evoked responses recorded from the human scalp. Electroencephalography and Clinical Neurophysiology, 28, 360–367.

Walter, W. G. (1967). Slow potential changes in the human brain associated with expectancy, decision and intention. Electroencephalography and Clinical Neurophysiology [Suppl.], 26, 123–130.

Walter, W. G., Cooper, R., Aldridge, V. J., McCallum, W. C., and Winter, A. L. (1964). Contingent negative variation: An electrical sign of sensori-motor association and expectancy in the human brain. Nature 203, 380–384.

Weerts, T., and Lang, P. (1973). The effects of eye fixation and stimulus and response location on the contingent negative variation (CNV). Biological Psychology, 1, 1–19.

Wiesendanger, M. (1981). Organization of secondary motor areas of cerebral cortex. In Brookhart, J. M., and Mountcastle, V. B. (Eds.), The nervous system, Vol. II, part 2 (pp. 1121–1147). Bethesda: American Physiological Society.

Weinberg, H., and Papakostopoulos, D. (1976). The frontal CNV: Its dissimilarity to CNVs recorded from other sites. Electroencephalography and Clinical Neurophysiology, 41, 476–482.

Wood, C. C., and Allison, T. (1981). Interpretation of evoked potentials: a neurophysiological perspective. Canadian Journal of Psychology, 35, 113–135.

Wood, C. C., Allison, T., Goff, W. R., Williamson. P.D., and Spencer, D. D. (1980). On the neural origin of P 300 in man. In H. H. Kornhuber and L. Deecke (Eds.), Motivation, motor and sensory processes of the brain: Electrical potentials, behaviour and clinical use. Progress in brain research, Vol. 54 (pp. 51–56). Amsterdam: Elsevier-North Holland Biomedical.

Speed-Accuracy Trade-offs in Motor Behavior: Theories of Impulse Variability

R. A. Schmidt, D. E. Sherwood, H. N. Zelaznik, and B. J. Leikind

Contents

Introduction

For centuries we have known that when people attempt to move quickly, they usually do so at the expense of spatial accuracy. Old statements such as "Haste makes waste" testify to the commonness of this kind of phenomenon. This effect is today termed the speed-accuracy trade-off, and has been the focus of considerable study in motor behavior. Until about six years ago, the general explanations of the speed-accuracy trade-off were in one way or another based on the idea

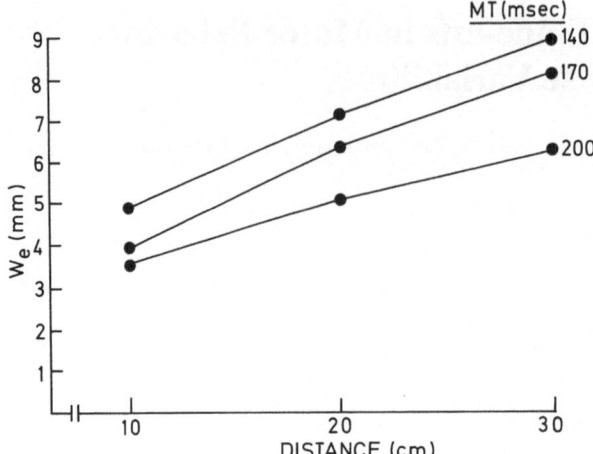

Fig. 1. The average within-subject SD of the movement endpoints (W_e) as a function of the movement distance (A) and the movement time (MT) in a single-aiming task. (From "Motor-output variability: A theory for the accuracy of rapid motor acts" by Schmidt, Zelaznik, Hawkins, Frank, and Quinn, *Psychological Review*, 1979, *86*, 415–451. Copyright 1979 by the American Psychological Association. Reprinted by permission of the publisher)

that when performers moved with a short movement time (MT) they reduced the time that was available for detecting errors in movement trajectory and for correcting them before the movement was completed. Hence, increases in MT lead to decreases in spatial error. These closed-loop explanations of the effect came in a variety of forms, and researchers have studied these speed-accuracy effects in a number of different paradigms (e.g., Crossman and Goodeve 1963, 1983; Fitts 1954; Howarth, Beggs, and Bowden 1971; Keele 1968).

In about 1977, a collection of people in our lab group (Schmidt, Zelaznik, and Frank 1978; Schmidt, Zelaznik, Hawkins, Frank, and Quinn 1979) began to doubt that these closed-loop explanations of the speed-accuracy effect were correct; at least we doubted whether *all* of the effect could be explained by feedback mechanisms. At the time, we were very interested in motor programming processes, with the notion that rapid movements appear to be structured in advance, and run off without much modification from ongoing feedback. We began to think of the speed-accuracy trade-off effects in these terms.

Initially, we were concerned with aiming tasks, where a hand-held stylus had to be moved a short distance to a target, with an MT that was reasonably short, less than 200 ms. These tasks seem to provide a nearly classical case of programmed actions. Yet, as we can see from Fig. 1, the speed-accuracy effect occurs very strongly here as well. In these data (Schmidt et al. 1979, Fig. 8), subjects were asked to move 10, 20, or 30 cm to a target, with MTs of 140, 170, or 200 ms. Clearly, as both MT decreased and movement amplitude (A) increased, errors (measured as the SD of the movement endpoints across trials, and labeled effective target width, W_e) increased systematically. If, as most would agree, feedback processes are probably minimal in these actions, how then, we asked, could the increases in error with decreases in *MT* be related to a decreased time for feedback processing? This basic question shifted our attention toward open-loop explanations of speed-accuracy effects and ultimately led to a model of them based on movement-output phenomena (Schmidt et al. 1978, 1979).

This chapter describes a set of our assumptions and other ideas that together constituted an impulse-variability theory for speed-accuracy trade-offs in rapid movements. Two different mathematical models of the trade-off effects have emerged. The initial paper by our group (Schmidt et al. 1979) provided one view, and another by Meyer, Smith, and Wright (1982), who were critical of our original mathematical modeling, provided a somewhat different one. These models rest on many of the same assumptions, and it is to these and the evidence for them that we turn first. We then discuss the actual modeling of these effects, first showing how we proceeded and then discussing some criticisms of these methods raised by Meyer et al. Next, we present some of the data from a variety of paradigms that support the predictions from both models. We then examine some problems with both models primarily in, but not limited to, the single-aiming paradigm. Our goal in this chapter is to provide a statement of the current status of impulse-variability modeling with respect to the viability of the assumptions, issues in modeling methods, and recent evidence. Later, we argue that these models seem to provide a good start in understanding speed-accuracy phenomena, but they are deficient in numerous ways. Some suggestions for future generations of these models are discussed.

An Impulse Model of Programming

We began with some of the general findings in the area of motor-programming research (see e.g., Schmidt 1982, 1984, for reviews), which suggested that motor programs produce *impulses* – that is, force integrated over time. This is not a particularly astounding idea, as just about all muscles can do is provide forces on bones through tendons.[1] These forces can be adjusted in amplitude by contracting the muscle at various tensions. Muscle timing, in terms of when a given muscle is active, how long it remains active, as well as the time course of that activity can also be under central motor-program control. This idea, referred to by some as the impulse-timing model of motor programming, makes specific predictions about how the pattern of muscular forces and their timing are altered as various aspects of a task are changed, e.g., as in aiming tasks when *A* and/or *MT* are altered.

Our choice to focus on impulses, rather than on any of a number of other physical quantities, was motivated by various factors. First, as already men-

---

[1] An acquaintance of one of us some years ago could propel a table tennis ball upward by placing it on the relaxed biceps muscle, then contracting the muscle sharply. But this is hardly a "natural" use of the musculature.

tioned, it seemed logical to assume that muscles produce impulses in their normal operation, and thus it seemed to be in keeping with a biological level of analysis. But second, impulses have some simple and interesting properties that make them appealing. One is that, from Newtonian kinematics, the velocity of an object (beginning at rest) after an impulse has stopped acting on it is directly proportional to the impulse size.

$$\text{Velocity} \propto \text{Impulse Size} \tag{1}$$

This statement is correct for force-time curves of *any* shape. More importantly from our perspective was the notion that the distance traveled by the time the impulse has stopped acting is directly proportional to the impulse size multiplied by the time over which it acts, provided that the "shape" or mathematical form of the force-time curve does not change as the impulse size changes (the *shape-constancy assumption*). If, for simplicity, we think of force-time curves as square waves, where the amplitude of the wave is F and its duration is t, and the force-time curve retains its form (here, as a square wave) as its force and duration change, we can say that the distance (d) traveled as a result of the impulse (again with the object beginning at rest) is given by

$$d \propto F \cdot t^2, \tag{2}$$

where the impulse size is $F \cdot t$. The generality of this relationship to the force-time curves typically found in movement situations – which are usually roughly sinusoidal in form, and clearly *not* square waves – is critically based on the shape-constancy assumption mentioned above.[2] We return to a discussion of the shape-constancy issue in a later section. For now, we can perhaps accept the view that impulses seem to provide a link with which to connect the programmed actions of the muscles and the movement trajectories that they ultimately produce in the limbs.

Generalized Motor Programs

Another important ingredient for our theorizing was a concept about how the pattern of forces (or impulses) is altered as the movement requirements affecting the speed-accuracy trade-off are changed, i.e., if the A and/or MT were altered. Some recent ideas provided at least one kind of answer for this question. A number of people (e.g., Pew 1974; Schmidt 1975, 1976) postulated that a given movement (e.g., an overarm throw or one's signature) may be based on a single

---

[2] In their critique of our model, Meyer et al. (1982) imply that we *assumed* that the force-time curves were square waves (e.g., their Figure 2 and p. 455), leaving the impression that we did not make a distinction between these and the sinusoid-like force-time functions that we usually see. Actually, we *modeled them as if* they were square waves, with the justification based on shape constancy and Equation 2. A proof of Equation 3 for sinusoidal force-time curves was given by Vaughn (personal communication) and for *any* form of force-time curve by Leikind (1985). A copy of the latter is in Appendix A.

underlying movement program, but that the resulting pattern could be expressed somewhat differently on different occasions by altering certain *parameters*. For example, a given pattern of action (one's signature is a good example) can be executed in a variety of ways, with a large or small size (check sized versus blackboard sized), rapidly or slowly, with great downward pressure or with a little, horizontally or vertically, etc. (see Merton 1974; Raibert 1977). It is also interesting to note that, when the signature is written on a check, the actions are made by the fingers, whereas with blackboard writing the action is done by the whole arm with the fingers being relatively fixed. All of this suggests that some underlying space-time pattern is represented, but that parameterizing the movement differently can result in different expressions of the "same" movement output. Space is not available here to discuss the evidence for this view in detail, but the interested reader could consult Schmidt (1982, in press) for a discussion of it. For the present purposes, the important idea is that a given motor program can be expressed in a variety of ways by making relatively simple transformations from the control signals to the musculature.

Invariance in Relative Timing

One can imagine a number of different versions of generalized motor program theory, each specifying which aspects of the movements are invariant and which can be easily varied to change the expression of the "same" movement. One version that was particularly influential to our thinking about speed-accuracy trade-offs held that an invariant feature of motor programs was *relative timing,* or the temporal structure of the impulses that defined a movement. Thus, when a given movement is produced more quickly, the motor system speeds up the entire sequence of impulses, but doing it in a way such that the relative timing is held invariant. That is, if one measures the duration (D_1) of an impulse in a certain action done in a certain movement time (MT_1), then when this movement is performed more rapidly on another occasion the duration of the analogous impulse (D_2) will be adjusted so that it is proportional to the new movement time (MT_2): thus, D_1/MT_1 should equal D_2/MT_2. Even though the relative timing may be unchanged, the amount of force produced in each impulse is easily changed from trial to trial. Thus, those of us who like to think in terms of generalized motor programs would say that relative timing is an invariant feature of the program, while overall force is a parameter (see Schmidt 1982, in press).

Generalized Motor Program Theory and Rapid Actions

Early in our thinking, we attempted to apply the notions in this version of generalized motor program theory – chiefly that relative timing was invariant and overall force and MT were parameters – to rapid limb actions where the speed-accuracy trade-off effects are most commonly seen. Consider one of the simplest

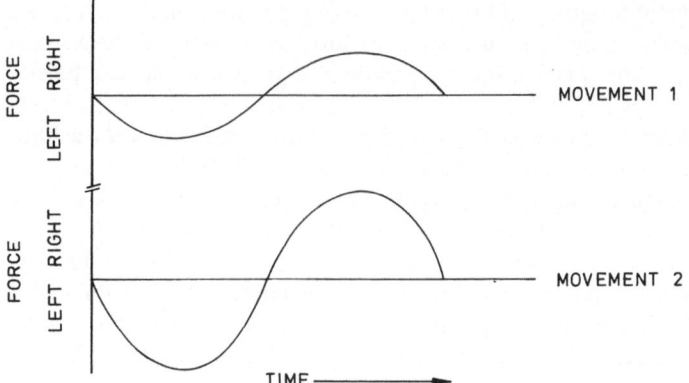

Fig. 2. Hypothetical force-time curves with Movement 1 having half the amplitude as Movement 2, but with the same *MT*. (From "Motor-output variability: A theory for the accuracy of rapid motor acts" by Schmidt, Zelaznik, Hawkins, Frank, and Quinn, *Psychological Review,* 1979, *86,* 415–451. Copyright 1979 by the American Psychological Association. Reprinted by permission of the publisher)

cases of these rapid actions, involving a task in which the subject must move a lever oriented in the horizontal plane from one position to another with an elbow flexion response, and so that the *MT* is close to some target value (say, 150 ms). An impulse for acceleration is produced in the direction of the target area which lasts about half the goal *MT*, and then another (for deceleration) is produced in the opposite direction that serves to slow the limb to bring it to a stop at or near a target. Figure 2 shows some idealized impulses that might come from such actions. What happens to the impulse as *A* is increased with the *MT* held constant? The theory says that the timing and "shape" of the impulses remains constant and only the amplitude of them is increased. If *A* is doubled, then the velocity at the end of the accelerative impulse must be doubled as well, and by Equation 1 the impulse size must be doubled. Thus, the motor system accomplishes this doubling in impulse size by doubling the height of the impulse with a constant duration and "shape." Thus, Movement 2 in Figure 2 would have twice the peak (or average) velocity as Movement 1, as its impulses are twice as large, and the limb would go twice as far in the same *MT*.

Figure 3 shows some actual force-time traces from such tasks in our laboratory (Shapiro and Walter 1984), with each trace being the average of approximately 20 responses. The different traces represent responses with the same *MT*, but with various *A*s. We can see that the force scales with *A*, but the duration of the impulses remains generally invariant. This is just the pattern of findings expected by the theory.

Next, consider what happens when *A* is fixed but the *MT* is varied. Here, the theory holds that the duration of each impulse should be proportional to *MT*, and that the impulse amplitude should be increased as the *MT* is decreased. Specifically, from Fig. 4 we see that as *MT* is halved the impulse durations are

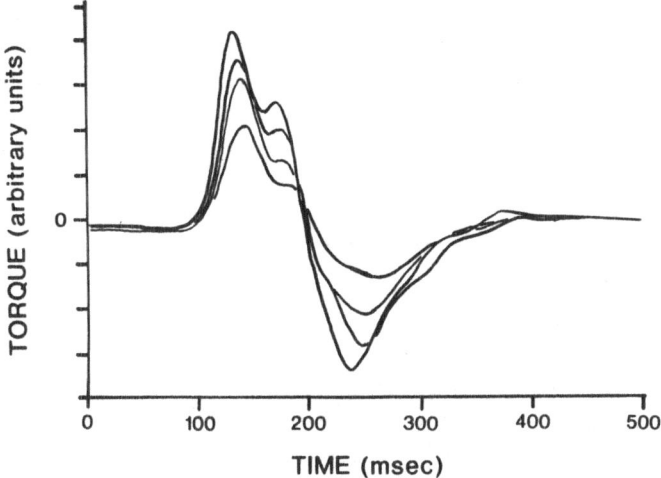

Fig. 3. Force-time curves from a rapid positioning task, where *MT* is fixed but *A* is varied experimentally in four steps. (Lengthening *A* results in systematically larger impulse amplitudes with an essentially constant impulse duration; from Shapiro and Walter 1984)

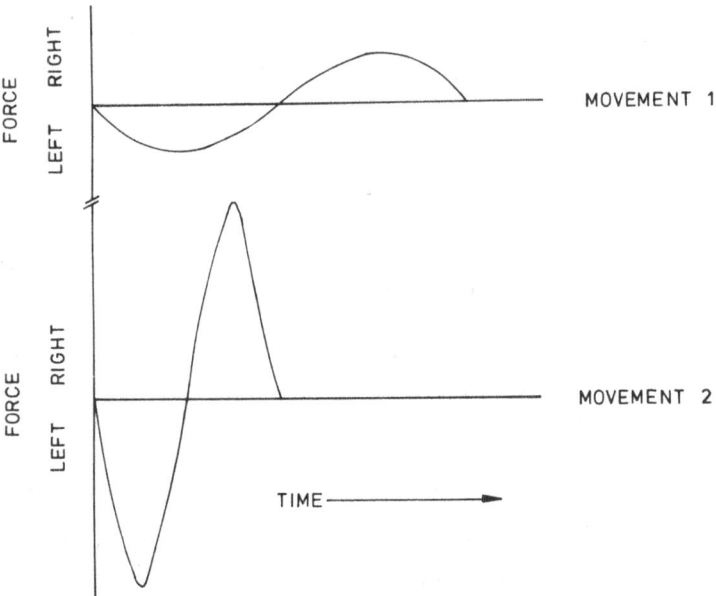

Fig. 4. Hypothetical force-time curves with Movement 1 having twice the *MT* as Movement 2, but with the same movement distance. (From "Motor-output variability: A theory for the accuracy of rapid motor acts" by Schmidt, Zelaznik, Hawkins, Frank, and Quinn, *Psychological Review,* 1979, *86,* 415–451. Copyright 1979 by the American Psychological Association. Reprinted by permission of the publisher)

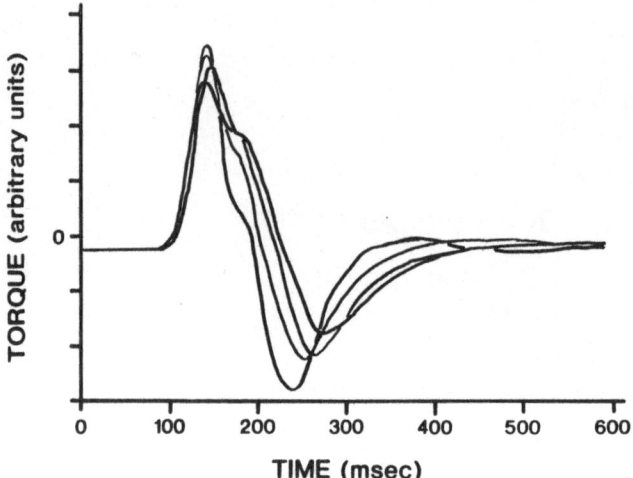

Fig. 5. Force-time curves in a rapid positioning task, where movement distance is fixed, but *MT* is varied experimentally in four steps. (Shortening the *MT* results in systematically larger forces and shorter impulse durations in both the agonist (upward) and antagonist (downward) phases of the responses; from Shapiro and Walter 1985)

halved, and the impulse amplitudes are increased by a factor of four; this extra force is necessary in order to provide twice the impulse (i.e., the area) needed to generate twice the average velocity (i.e., the same distance in half the time).

In Fig. 5 are another set of force-time curves from Shapiro and Walter (1984), this time for situations in which the *MT* is varied from 150 to 270 ms while *A* is fixed. Here, the impulse durations change markedly with *MT*. The shortest *MT*s are associated with the largest forces, but the relative amplitudes are not quite as the theory would expect. The theory does seem to predict the temporal structure relatively well, however.

What do these changes in impulse duration with *MT* mean for conceptualizations of the generalized motor program? On the one hand, they might simply mean that whenever the *MT* is changed, successfully accomplishing the goal of moving the same distance in a smaller *MT* essentially requires (from Newtonian kinematics) that the impulses behave as shown in Figs. 4 and 5; this evidence might not say much about how the motor program is modified to achieve this goal. But a number of authors (e.g., Carter and Shapiro, in press; Shapiro and Walter 1984) have shown that such changes in the kinetics (forces) of movements with *MT* can, under at least some circumstances, be closely related to the changes in EMGs, implying that these changes in impulse duration here are indeed a part of the control signal to the muscles.

An additional set of data from our laboratory show this particularly well. We (Schmidt, Sherwood, and Walter 1985 b) used a "reversal task" in which the subject flexed the elbow to move a horizontal lever to a target area 45° away, reversed direction, and then followed through past the original starting point, with

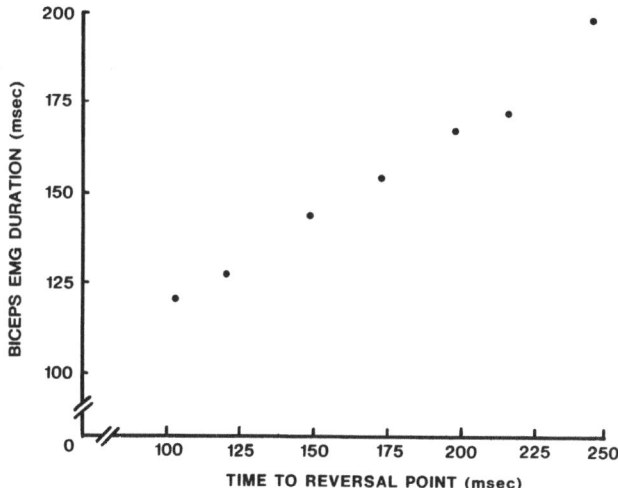

Fig. 6. Biceps EMG duration as a function of the time to the reversal point in rapid reversal responses. (From Schmidt et al. 1985 b)

the requirement that the total time from movement initiation until the limb passed the starting point be close to some goal *MT* (e.g., 200 ms). We recorded the EMGs from the biceps and triceps muscles, and measured the durations of the bursts as a function of the goal time to the reversal point set by the experimenter. This time to reversal ranged from essentially the subject's minimum (or 100 ms to reversal) in 25-ms steps up to 250 ms to reversal. The biceps EMG durations are shown in Fig. 6. There was a clear linear trend for the biceps EMG duration to decrease with decreases in *MT*, even down to the shortest time to reversal possible. To us, this suggests that the control signal from the spinal cord to the musculature modulates impulse durations when *MT*s are changed, and thus the changes in the limb's impulse characteristics are indicative of the ways in which the various muscles are controlled by the program.

To summarize briefly, initially we had a number of ideas about how the control signals to the musculature in rapid limb action would be modified as the characteristics of the movement to be made were changed (e.g., longer *A* or shorter *MT*). These ideas have been supported recently by a considerable body of experimental data, which adds to our current confidence in them, but the original ideas on which the theory was based were at the time considerably more speculative. The next concern was to take these views about impulses and motor-program functioning, and to try to generate an explanation of the speed-accuracy trade-off. We began by assuming that the impulses produced by the program were variable (within subjects, across trials of the "same" task) and that the sources of this variability and its magnitude depended strongly on the variables like *A* and *MT*. We turn to these issues next.

The Impulse-Variability Model

We were interested in understanding the errors involved in the goal achievement in simple motor tasks as a function of the impulses that were driving the limb. Error in such tasks can be measured in many ways, but certainly chief among them is variable error or the variability (SD) of the subject's responses about his or her own mean. For this reason, we sought sources of *variability* in the impulses that produce the spatial variabilities in the movement endpoint, hoping to be able to relate the two in some way. The idea was simple: Impulses cause movement and determine trajectories; thus, variability in impulses should lead to variability in trajectories, and hence to variabilities in movement endpoint, which is our measure of error.

The theory holds that, when the subject's goal is constant (i.e., fixed A and MT), then over trials the impulse size will be variable about the subject's mean impulse for that A-MT combination. Further, this variability can be analyzed, according to our view, into two separate and independent sources: (a) variability in the force dimension of the impulse and (b) variability in the duration over which the force acts. The division of impulse inconsistency into force and time variability has been a reasonable one, but the notion of the *independence* of these sources of variability has been challenged recently (e.g., Newell, Carlton, and Carlton 1982; Sherwood 1983). We will discuss implications of this assumption in a later section.

Sources of Variability

We next asked how these sources of variability were related to the independent variables of major interest here – A and MT. We knew that as A increases or MT decreases, errors increase (Fig. 1). Also, these changes imply increases in force produced, and thus we began to ask about how force and the *variability in force* were related. If force variability should increase with force, and more force is required when MT is decreased and/or A is increased, then the resulting increases in impulse variability could, perhaps, explain how these changes in A or MT can predict errors.

Force variability. We were unable to find data in the literature that related force and force variability, and so we (Schmidt et al. 1978, 1979) and later a number of others (Newell et al. 1982; Sherwood and Schmidt 1980) conducted a series of experiments seeking to determine the nature of this relationship. Typically, subjects were asked to make ballistic (non-feedback-based) contractions of the elbow flexors to "shoot" a dot on an oscilloscope screen to a target. The amount of force could be varied between blocks by changing the height of the target, and subjects made a series of about 40 contractions, for each of which the goal was to make the peak force achieve the given target level. The contractions occurred about one per second in time to a metronome. We were interested in the within-subject SD of these peak forces as a function of the amount of force required.

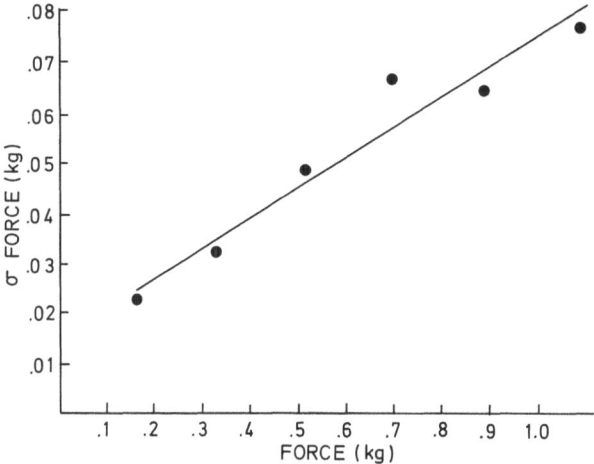

Fig. 7. Relationship between force and force variability in elbow flexion responses. (From "Motor-output variability: A theory for the accuracy of rapid motor acts" by Schmidt, Zelaznik, Hawkins, Frank, and Quinn, *Psychological Review,* 1979, *86,* 415–451. Copyright 1979 by the American Psychological Association. Reprinted by permission of the publisher)

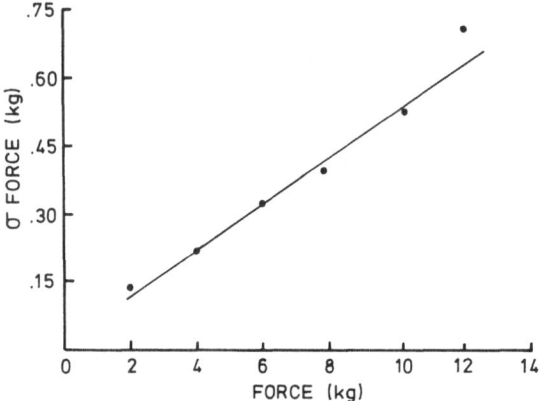

Fig. 8. Relationship between force and force variability in elbow flexion responses (the forces produced are far larger than in Fig. 7). (From "Motor-output variability: A theory for the accuracy of rapid motor acts" by Schmidt, Zelaznik, Hawkins, Frank, and Quinn, *Psychological Review,* 1979, *86,* 415–451. Copyright 1979 by the American Psychological Association. Reprinted by permission of the publisher`

Some of our findings are shown in Figs. 7 and 8. In Fig. 7, where the forces were quite small, a generally linear relationship emerged between force and force variability. The forces were much larger in the data shown in Fig. 8, but the same overall linear relationship was evidenced, although here the slope was somewhat smaller. Generally, from a number of our experiments on this issue, we argued that force and force variability were roughly linearly related, with the relationship being almost proportional up to about 65% of the subject's maximum force.

SD (force) $\propto$ force   (3)

We also noticed that, as the sizes of the forces required in our various experiments became larger, the slope of the linear relationship generally decreased, suggesting that the "true" relationship between force and force variability may be slightly curvilinear (concave downward) rather than strictly linear. Nevertheless, in our modeling efforts, it was much simpler to consider the force-variability/force relationship as being linear, and this was the relationship used in our model (Schmidt et al. 1978, 1979) and in that by Meyer et al. (1982).

In modeling, we and others (Meyer et al. 1982) have for simplicity considered that force variability and force were proportional – i.e., that the relationship was linear with a zero intercept. We have always found small, perhaps negligible, nonzero intercepts in our data, with the size of the intercept tending to decrease as the sizes of the forces studied decreased. But these relationships have been determined on relatively narrow ranges of forces in each experiment, and Newell et al. (1982) and Newell, Carlton, and Hancock (in press) have shown that the force-variability function over the entire range of forces is concave downward as we suspected, curving gently upward from the origin; the intercept of the function is probably very close to zero. It is arguable as to whether this intercept could ever be exactly zero in practice, however, as the smallest possible contraction is that produced by a single motor unit, below which no values will lie on the actual force-variability/force function.

After our model was published, we continued to examine the force-variability/force relationship with somewhat larger forces, with some forces approaching the subject's maximum. One of our studies (Sherwood and Schmidt 1980) showed an inverted-U relationship. The force variability increased roughly linearly (as we had found before) up to about 65% of the subject's maximum, but then force variability decreased as the force requirements were increased further (Fig. 9). In that paper, we reported the same general effect for dynamic (shortening) contractions. While these results may, at first glance, seem surprising, they are perhaps best seen as the result of a natural limitation on variability when the maximum force is approached. When the required contraction is, say, 99% of maximum, there is little "room for" variability above this value, and hence vari-

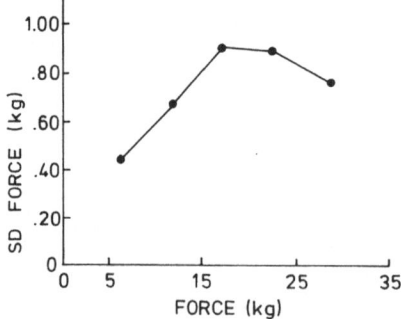

Fig. 9. The average within-subject SD of the peak force produced as a function of the force produced. (Forces were considerably larger than in Fig. 8; from Sherwood and Schmidt 1980)

ability will be reduced by this ceiling effect. We will discuss the implications of this finding for the speed-accuracy trade-off effect in a later section (pages 108–112).

Not everyone has found these inverted-U effects, and there has emerged a minor controversy about them. Newell et al. (1982) have shown a generally continuously increasing (negatively accelerated) force variability as a function of force in dynamic contractions, but the movements they have used resulted in only 68% of the subject's maximum force, just about where Sherwood and Schmidt (1980) found the peak in force variability to lie (Fig. 9). Also, Newell et al. show trends toward this inverted-U relationship, especially in their conditions where the lever to be moved was loaded with an additional mass (see Newell et al. 1982, Figs. 5f–j), although they chose not to emphasize this aspect of their data. Further, Newell and Carlton (1983) and Newell et al. (in press) have shown rather convincingly that the form of the relationship between force variability and force depends on the rate of rise of force within the contractions. If the subjects increase their time to peak force as the force requirements become very large, then this could explain why force variability decreases past about 65% of maximum in our data. Thus it may be that the inverted-U function that Sherwood and Schmidt (1980) have found is more related to strategies in producing force than it is to any inherent characteristic of the neuromuscular system. Indeed, in one of our recent studies with reversal tasks, we (Sherwood, Schmidt, and Walter 1985) show that when the time to peak force is controlled by holding MT constant and changing A, the inverted-U form is not present even with relatively large forces, but rather force variability increases monotonically with increased force.

Finally, a few years after we presented our data on force and force variability, it came to our attention that many of these questions had been asked before. In a fine review of the topic, Newell et al. (in press) cite some very old literature on this issue, in which it was found that force variability generally increases as force increases, but with a decreasing slope and no inverted-U (Fullerton and Cattell 1892; Jenkins 1947; Noble and Bahrick 1956; Woodworth 1901). While these experiments generally show the kinds of force-variability functions that we found later – except for the inverted-U relationships – they do not quite give the information we needed to know for use in conjunction with the impulse-variability notions. The major problem is that these earlier experiments used very slow contractions, where adjustments in forces were permitted within each, and some (e.g., Fullerton and Cattell 1892) confounded force with distance moved. From the point of view of impulse-variability theory, the interest was in totally preprogrammed forces, made quickly without possibility of subsequent adjustments, so that the relationship between what was programmed and the movement that resulted could be studied. Had we known about these studies, our job would have been much easier, but it is now clear that most of our rapid-contraction work would have been done in any case. But the early experiments do remind us of an old idea in science: If you think you have found something new, you probably just haven't done your homework.

In summary, many separate experiments have shown a roughly linear, or slightly curvilinear (concave downward), relationship between force variability and force, strongly suggesting that the speed–accuracy relationships may be based in part on the tendency of the motor system to produce more force inconsistency as force requirements are increased. In modeling, both Schmidt et al. (1978, 1979) and Meyer et al. (1982) have used a rather idealized statement of this relationship, where force variability is regarded as proportional to force. Recent evidence showing curvilinearity in this relation, showing nonzero intercepts, and showing inverted-U relationships at very large forces, leads to serious concerns about modeling force variability in the way we and others have.

Temporal variability. Impulse variability, as we (Schmidt et al. 1978, 1979) viewed it, is the result of an additional source of variability – the variability in the *duration* of the impulse. Our view of the control of impulses held that the central nervous system in some way controls the duration over which a muscle is excited, and thus the duration of the impulse caused by it. If the impulse duration can be viewed as the result of some time-production system (or oscillator) "in" the central nervous system, then this system should behave in ways similar to other time-production systems that have been studied in the past. In tapping tasks, for example, it has generally been found that as the duration of the interval to be produced increases there is an increase in the variability of these intervals (Michon 1967; Wing and Kristofferson 1973). The exact form of this increase seems to be different for different paradigms, so for application to our own modeling problem we studied impulse durations and their variabilities as a function of the length of the impulse duration in rapid limb movements. We varied

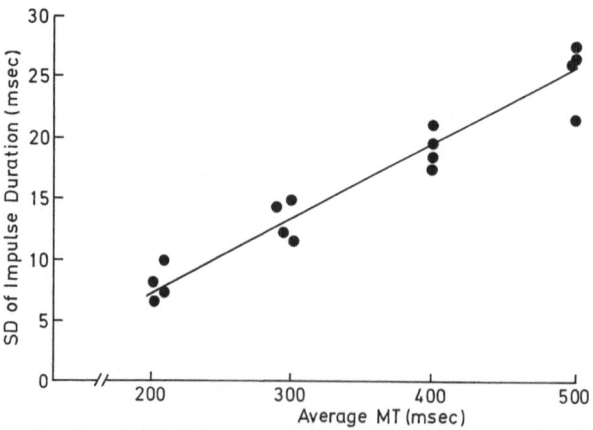

Fig. 10. Variability in impulse duration in a reciprocal movement task as a function of the instructed *MT*. (From "Motor-output variability: A theory for the accuracy of rapid motor acts" by Schmidt, Zelaznik, Hawkins, Frank, and Quinn, *Psychological Review*, 1979, *86*, 415–451. Copyright 1979 by the American Psychological Association. Reprinted by permission of the publisher)

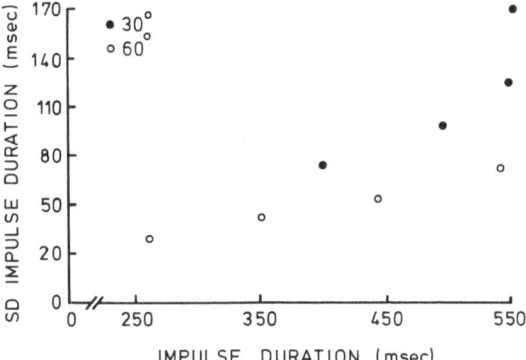

Fig. 11. Variability in impulse duration in a ballistic timing task as a function of the impulse duration. (From Sherwood 1983)

experimentally the duration of the impulse by altering the *MT*, and studied the variability in the impulse duration as a function of it.

In one experiment (Schmidt et al., Fig. 4), we asked subjects to move a lever back and forth between two targets in time to a metronome, without making corrections at each endpoint. The *MT* was varied between sessions by the metronome setting, so that *MT*s of 200, 300, 400, and 500 ms/half-cycle were produced. We also studied movement distance (16°, 32°, 48°, and 64°), crossed experimentally with the four *MT*s, with each of the 16 combinations in a different session. The forces applied to the lever handle were recorded, and the durations of the impulses for each of about 40 oscillations were measured. The SD of these impulse durations was the measure of primary interest. Fig. 10 shows that, as the *MT* (and the impulse duration) increased, there was a generally linear increase in impulse duration variability, and this relation was essentially independent of the four movement distances (seen as the four points at each *MT* condition).

Later, Sherwood (1983) examined this relationship in discrete tasks where subjects were asked to move either 30° or 60° to pass through a switch such that the *MT* was close to some goal *MT* (e.g., 150 ms), a task many have referred to as *ballistic timing*. Sherwood's data are shown in Fig. 11. For each of the movement distances, there was a generally linear increase in the SD of the impulse durations as the impulse duration increased (manipulated by altering the instructed *MT* experimentally). This relationship was very strong for the 60° movements where the impulses were large and well defined, but less strong for the 30° movements. Sherwood argued that the data point at the upper right, representing the slowest movement condition, should not be considered, as the EMGs and impulses did not show the typical agonist-antagonist pattern found in the other movement conditions. If this data point is ignored, then the linear relationship between impulse duration and its SD is again supported for conditions which satisfy the assumptions of the model (ballistic, rapid actions). This is an important point, as it illustrates one difficulty we and others have had in studying impulse-variability phenomena. If the movements studied do not conform to the assumptions underlying the impulse-variability model, then the impulse-variability model cannot be expected to predict well.

Thus, the earlier work on time-interval production has suggested, and our work with impulses in various movement situations has generally shown, that as the *MT* (and hence the impulse duration) increases, there is a generally linear increase in the SD of the impulse duration. In our data on impulses (Fig. 10) that led to the impulse-variability model, this relationship appeared to be linear and nearly proportional, and so for simplicity we argued that the variability of the impulse duration should be proportional to impulse duration.

SD (impulse duration) $\propto$ impulse duration   (4)

Subsequent data (e.g., in Fig. 11) suggest that the relationship is not quite proportional. As with the relationships between force and its variability, future impulse variability models will surely benefit from further attempts to describe the relationship between impulse duration and its variability, which is probably not as simple as we have characterized it in Equation 4.

The Shape-Constancy Assumption

Both the Schmidt et al. (1979) and Meyer et al. (1982) models of impulse variability are critically dependent on the notion that the mathematical form, or "shape," of the impulse remains fixed as the size of the impulse varies with *A* and/or *MT*. Recall that Leikind (1985) had shown that Equation 2, which expresses the distance traveled as a function of impulse size, was correct only if shape constancy held. We turn now to a brief discussion of this important issue.

First, a more formal definition: Two impulses have the same shape if and only if their amplitudes, measured at the same *relative* time, are proportional. If one chooses *any* pair of relative times through an impulse – say, .40 and .80 of the impulse duration – then for the impulses to have the same shape the impulses must have heights (forces) that are directly proportional to each other at these points. That is, the ratio of forces computed at .40 for the two impulses should be equal to the ratio of the forces computed at .80. And, this relationship must hold for *any* proportions of impulse duration chosen. This mathematical restriction means that, as the impulse grows in size (with changes in *A* or *MT*, for example), it grows by proportional "stretching" along the time and/or force dimensions, such that the overall form remains constant. (See also Meyer et al. 1982, who discuss this issue in terms of force-parameter and time-function rescalability.)

To what extent does this assumption of shape constancy hold for impulses driving movements of interest here? Early in our work on this problem, we suspected that such a principle might be at least roughly correct, bolstered by the findings from Denier van der Gon and Thuring (1965), Armstrong (1970), and Shapiro (1977) that the *space*-time patterns tend to maintain their shapes under changes in various movement parameters. If the *force*-time pattern retains its shape as the space-time pattern appears to do, then this would be evidence for a shape constancy. Hollerbach (1981) did provide some data showing that acceleration-time patterns generally tended to hold their shape in the face of changes in amplitude of handwriting; but even so, the evidence for shape constancy when we published our 1979 model was very sketchy indeed.

Since then, we have examined this question in somewhat more detail. Shapiro and Walter (1984) and Sherwood (1983) examined various discrete lever-movement tasks as a function of A and MT, where forces were measured during the movement via a strain gauge. Some of the records from Shapiro and Walter are shown in Fig. 3 (changes in A with MT constant) and Fig. 5 (changes in MT with A constant). From these figures, and from analogous kinds of analyses done by Sherwood (1983), one does receive the impression that the shape-constancy assumption is at least roughly correct. But these shapes have not been measured in detail, and it is doubtful as to whether these data would support a strict interpretation of shape constancy such as we have discussed here. Some more detailed analyses of the shape-constancy assumption are being conducted at present by one of us (D.E.S.), but the methods are still being worked out and it is somewhat too early to predict the outcome. But, we have the general impression that, in these tasks at least, the shape-constancy assumption is not seriously violated.

A somewhat more systematic probe into shape constancy in aiming tasks has been undertaken by us in conjunction with Stan Gielen at the University of Utrecht. In two separate studies, we examined the acceleration-time functions in three-dimensional stylus-aiming tasks, in which the subject had to move from a home position to a target in a specified MT. In one experiment (Zelaznik and Schmidt 1983), the movement was photographed with infrared light-sensitive film, and an LED attached to the stylus was pulsed every 10 ms; the stylus positions as a function of time were later hand-digitized, and the resulting function differentiated twice after smoothing to obtain the horizontal and vertical acceleration-time functions. In the other experiment (Schmidt, Gielen, and Zelaznik 1985 a), the aiming task was filmed from above via a Selspot system, with the position of the stylus in the horizontal dimension being measured by computer every 3 ms. The position-time functions were smoothed and differentiated twice to obtain acceleration-time functions. In the first experiment, we studied the aiming task under three different As (10, 20, and 30 cm) and three different MTs (150, 200, and 250 ms). In the second experiment, the A was fixed at 20 cm, but the MT was varied in five steps (125, 150, 175, 200, and 225 ms).

The averaged horizontal acceleration time functions for the three MTs of one subject in the Zelaznik-Schmidt study are shown in Fig. 12. (The results are near-ly identical in both studies.) In the figure, acceleration toward (up) and away from (down) the target are presented as a function of *relative* time through the movement; for example, the value of 50% on the abscissa means that one-half of the instructed MT had elapsed for each of the movements being plotted. The shape-constancy assumption demands that, with the accelerations plotted in rela-tive time as they are here, the various "landmarks" such as peak acceleration,

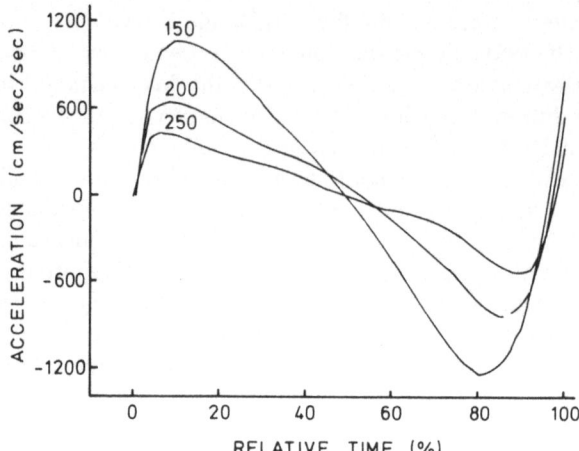

Fig. 12. Horizontal acceleration-time functions, plotted in terms of relative time, from 30-cm single-aiming movements. (The MTs were 150, 200, and 250 ms; from Zelaznik and Schmidt 1983)

time of return to zero acceleration, and peak deceleration should line up nearly perfectly. We can see clearly from the figure that with changes in MT there is a marked shift in relative time of appearance of the peak acceleration, with the peak acceleration occurring later (in relative time) as the MT decreases. Similarly, the peak deceleration occurs relatively earlier as the MT decreases. It seems clear that the accelerations do not scale in relative time as the shape-constancy assumption demands.

These effects can be viewed in somewhat more detail in other ways. In Fig. 13, various measures taken from the acceleration-time curves are plotted as a function of the goal MT. First, consider the time from the beginning of the movement until peak acceleration (*peak positive* in the figure). If the shape-constancy assumption holds, then time to peak acceleration should be proportional to MT. But from Fig. 13, we see that it is essentially constant, with no effects of either A or MT. This rather constant time to peak acceleration is similar to that reported by Ghez (1979) and Ghez and Vicario (1978). A similar picture emerges if we consider the interval from the peak deceleration until the end of the movement (*peak negative*), as it is nearly constant and considerably longer than the time to peak acceleration. These measures show that the initial portions of acceleration and the final portions of deceleration do not scale with MT and that the shape-constancy assumption is seriously violated. On the other hand, the duration of acceleration (*positive* in the figure) and the duration of deceleration (*negative*) both scale with MT as of course they must. Further, it is evident that the amount of time involved in deceleration is considerably greater than the time in acceleration, and thus the acceleration-time function is not symmetrical in time.

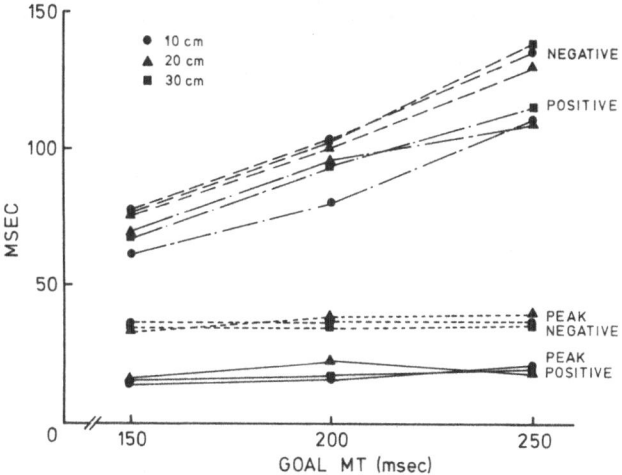

Fig. 13. The durations of various parameters of acceleration-time functions from single-aiming movements. (*peak positive* is the interval from movement initiation to peak positive acceleration, and *peak negative* is the interval from peak deceleration to the end of movement. *Negative* and *positive* are durations of negative and positive acceleration respectively; from Zelaznik and Schmidt 1983)

These data provide strong implications for impulse-variability models. Both the Schmidt et al. (1978, 1979) model and the Meyer et al. (1982) model rest strongly on the shape-constancy assumption. Yet, in one of the most important movement paradigms for which an explanation of the speed-accuracy relationship is offered – the single-aiming paradigm – the shape-constancy assumption appears not to be correct. To the extent that these deviations from shape constancy produce major differences in the actual versus expected movement trajectories, the models will surely be in error with respect to the predicted effects of A and MT. Furthermore, the Meyer et al. model, which they term the *symmetrical* impulse-variability model, demands that the acceleration-time functions be symmetrical – i.e., the accelerative impulse should be an inverted mirror image of the decelerative impulse. (The Schmidt et al. model has no such requirement.) The data here show that the accelerative impulse is both shorter in absolute time and larger in amplitude than the decelerative impulse and thus shows serious departures from the symmetricality expected by Meyer et al.

Finally, it should be mentioned that Meyer et al. (1982, p. 474) have abandoned the notion of temporal rescalability for one of the paradigms under consideration here – the ballistic-timing task. Instead, they have the *temporal* structure of the acceleration-time function fixed at its longest duration and then account for the subject's variations in MT by modifying the amplitude of the function to generate larger or smaller initial impulses. But this assumption seems contradictory to a number of our results. A fixed temporal structure implies that measures such as the time to peak acceleration should also be invariant as MT is changed experimentally, as indeed should *all* of the temporal "landmarks." But

Sherwood (1983) with ballistic timing found that the time to peak acceleration systematically increased as MT increased (176, 211, 243, and 270 ms for instructed MTs of 150, 200, 250, and 300 ms).[3] And, the relative time to peak acceleration (or the time to peak divided by the total impulse duration) was nearly constant (54%, 50%, 49%, and 49%, respectively) for the four MTs as would be expected from an acceleration-time rescaling in the temporal dimension. This assumption underlying the modeling of ballistic-timing tasks in Meyer et al.'s model seems clearly incorrect to us.

To summarize, the critical shape-constancy assumption of the impulse-variability models of Schmidt et al. (1978, 1979) and Meyer et al. (1982) have only mixed support. Superficial analyses of some movement situations, to date involving either slower sequential movements (e.g., handwriting, lever movements) or somewhat more rapid single-joint movements, appear to show roughly constant acceleration-time function shapes as A or MT are varied. Yet, in more rapid three-dimensional movements (e.g., single-aiming, Figs. 12, 13) this shape-constancy assumption is rather seriously violated. Whether this difference is due to (a) rapid versus slow movements, (b) one-dimensional versus three-dimensional movements, or (c) to other differences between these movement categories that have not been identified will have to await further experimentation. But for now, it appears that future impulse-variability models should not rely on this questionable assumption.

Modeling Impulse Variability

Both the Schmidt et al. (1978, 1979) and Meyer et al. (1982) models have used the assumptions mentioned in the previous sections (symmetricality is the single exception) to derive the expected effects of changes in A and/or MT on the impulse variability. Even though these models rest on nearly identical bases, additional assumptions are made by each, and there are considerable differences in the mathematics used to provide the derivations. In this section, we first describe our original view of modeling for impulse variability, as it provides (we think) a useful way to conceptualize the problem. We then turn to some criticisms of these methods raised by Meyer et al.

Equations 3 and 4 provide the basic starting point (together with the assumptions listed previously) for modeling impulse variability, as they describe how we and Meyer et al. thought that the components of impulse variability change as certain features of the movement (i.e., A and/or MT) change. Figure 14 shows two sets of idealized impulses from two movements, with the "taller" impulse in each set representing a movement with half the MT of the "shorter" one. These impulses are diagrammed as square waves for simplicity in

---

[3] The times to peak acceleration are approximately equal to, and occasionally even shorter than, the MT because of the long-duration follow-through past the switch that defines the end of MT.

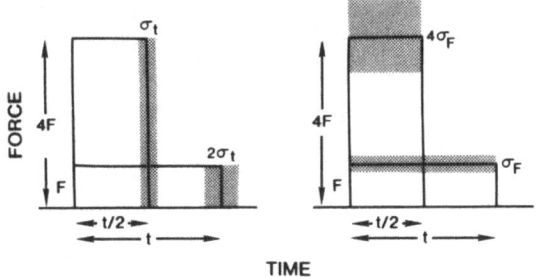

TIME

Fig. 14. The modeling of the temporal components of impulse variability (*left*) and the force components of impulse variability (*right*), shown as *shaded areas*. (Each pair of agonist force-time curves represents two movements, one with half the *MT* of the other)

explanation, although any form of these functions could have been used given the shape-constancy assumption.[4] The left pair of figures is drawn under the temporary restriction that there is no variability in force, which allows us to examine the relationship between *MT* and the temporal component of impulse variability, shown as the shaded areas. The pair of figures on the right involves the opposite restriction, wherein no variability in the temporal component of the impulses is assumed, with the effects of *MT* on the force components being considered. We turn to an analysis of each of these cases next.

Temporal variability. From Equation 4, as the *MT* decreases, the temporal variability decreases proportionally. But, the shaded *area* (i.e., the impulse variability) is the product of a temporal variability that is halved and a force that is increased by a factor of four. That is, temporal variability for the longer *MT* is $2 \, \sigma_t \times F = 2 \, \sigma_t F$, whereas the analogous component of variability for the shorter *MT* is $\sigma_t \times 4 \, F = 4 \, \sigma_t F$. In this case, halving the *MT* has resulted in the portion of impulse variability attributable to variations in time to be doubled, from $2 \, \sigma_t F$ to $4 \, \sigma_t F$. Generally, the temporal component of the impulse variability is directly proportional to $1/MT$. It is also directly proportional to A, since force increases linearly with A while the impulse duration (and hence the impulse-duration variability) is constant. Combining these two factors yields the result that the temporal component of variability is directly proportional to A/MT.

Force variability. Next, consider the curves to the right of Fig. 14, where no temporal variability is assumed. In this case, as the *MT* is halved, the amount of force, and thus the amount of force variability (from Equation 3), is increased by a factor of four. But the impulse variability (the shaded area) is represented as a force variability four times as large multiplied by an impulse duration that is halved, so that the impulse variability is doubled as the *MT* is halved. That is, the

---

[4] Our present knowledge that the shape-constancy assumption may not be correct at least for aiming responses (Zelaznik and Schmidt 1983) argues against this approach to the problem.

impulse variability for the longer MT is $\sigma_f \times t = \sigma_f t$, while the impulse variability for the shorter MT is $4\,\sigma_f \times t/2 = 2\,\sigma_f t$. Generally, the force variability component of impulse variability is related to $1/MT$, just as the temporal component is. Also, the force-variability component is directly related to A, since the variability in force would increase directly with A, with the impulse duration fixed. Combining these two factors yields the result that the variability in the force component of the impulse is related to A/MT, again just as the temporal component is.

Force and time variability. From the above two informal arguments, the relationship between the temporal and force components of variability considered in isolation are the same – i.e., both are directly proportional to A/MT. If we make the assumption that these two sources of variability are independent, then their joint effects (expressed as variances) when both are allowed to vary can be thought of as the sum of both components. Since both effects separately are the same, then total impulse variability should be related to A/MT.

Impulse variability $\propto$ A/MT. (5)

And, because the velocity of an object after the impulse has stopped acting on it is proportional to impulse size, it follows that

Velocity variability $\propto$ A/MT. (6)

These basic relationships, connecting the variability in the velocity of an object, the impulse size, and A/MT are the cornerstone of our model. Presumably, if each muscle in a complex movement produces impulses each of whose variability is proportional to A/MT, then the *ensemble* of muscular impulses should also follow the same principles.

Criticisms of Our Modeling Procedures

A number of criticisms of the ways we modeled impulse variability can be raised, some of which were also pointed out by Meyer et al. (1982). We will deal with three of these problems here and leave the remaining ones for a subsequent section (pages 114–115).

Independence of force variability and temporal variability. One difficulty is that our derivations require that force variability and time variability be statistically independent, an assumption needed in order to treat the two sources of variability as additive. Specifically, this means that, for a single subject performing under a given A/MT combination, and where the subject's intended A and MT are constant across trials, the agonist impulse duration and agonist impulse amplitude will be correlated zero. This should not be confused with the situation where the subject's intended A and MT are allowed to change between trials; here impulse duration and amplitude will change systematically, and in tight inverse relationship to each other (as described earlier). Force and time variability should be substantially negatively correlated in this case.

Initially, we had some reason to suspect that force and time variability might be independent as defined above. At least, if some correlation occurred between them, we guessed that it would be small and would not materially affect the accuracy of our predictions. We may have been wrong. Subsequent to work on our model, Newell et al. (1982) and Sherwood (1983) provided evidence that the correlation between impulse amplitude and impulse duration in various movement tasks ranged from about −.2 to −.6 and that the correlation seemed to increase slightly (in the negative direction) as the impulse size increased. Sherwood (1983, 1984) has argued that the existence of the nonzero correlation between impulse duration and impulse amplitude per se does not affect our derivations, as it only requires a change in the slope of the function relating A/MT to impulse variability, while retaining its critical linearity. But the finding that the correlation increases (in the negative direction) with increases in impulse size does provide further difficulties, as it predicts a negatively accelerating relationship between A/MT and impulse variability. These effects of the changing correlation should be recognized in future modeling efforts.

Probability theory. Meyer et al. have argued that we modeled the sources of variability improperly and that our Equation 8 (in Schmidt et al. 1979) should have stated that the variability in the impulse was proportional to $1/MT$ rather than to $1/MT^2$. Meyer et al. are correct here. We should have said that the variability in the *force component* of the impulse was related to $1/MT^2$. However, analyzing as we did the variability in the force *component* (proportional to $1/MT^2$) and the variability in the temporal *component* (proportional to MT), we come to the same conclusion as Meyer et al., namely that variability in the impulse is related to $1/MT$. Thus, there is really no disagreement about the nature of this relationship shown here as Equation 5.

Additivity of sources of variability. Meyer et al. (1982, Footnote 5) also criticized our method of considering separately the force and temporal components of variability. As described above, we temporarily held one constant while considering variability in the other and then added their separate effects when both were allowed to vary freely. Meyer et al. stated that the only time such procedures are valid is if the SD $(F \cdot T) \propto$ SD $(F) \cdot$ SD (t). But, under the assumptions of our model – namely (a) that SD $(F) \propto F$ and SD $(t) \propto t$, (b) that F and t are independent for a given movement goal, and (c) that SD (F) and SD (t) are "reasonably small" (Duncan 1952) – this is precisely the relationship that we show to hold in Appendix A (Equation A5). We feel that this criticism of our methods was not warranted.

Some Tests of the Major Assumptions

In this section, we examine the evidence for some of the major assumptions and predictions from the impulse-variability idea. Some of these are fundamental to

the basic ideas of the model, as they deal with the variability in velocity produced by an impulse as a function of certain variables that affect impulse size.
Others are predictions from the model as it applies to the performance of certain
movement tasks. In both cases, there is reasonably good agreement between the
predictions and the empirical evidence, as we shall see next.

Velocity and Impulse Size

Absolutely fundamental to any model attempting to relate kinematics of movements to impulses is the notion that impulse size and the velocity that results
from that impulse are tightly related. This relationship is summarized in Equation 1, where from elementary Newtonian kinematics the velocity of an object by
the time an impulse has ceased acting on it (assuming it began with zero velocity)
is directly proportional to the impulse size. Recently, Sherwood (1983, 1984) has
evaluated this assumption by having subjects make horizontal ballistic-timing responses involving a lever. The action began with the lever against a stop, and
then the subject moved through either 30° or 60° past a switch, with a follow-
through beyond the switch allowed and encouraged. Subjects performed in four
MT conditions – 150, 200, 250, and 300 ms, in separate blocks of trials. Impulses
were measured via a strain gauge attached to the handle the subject grasped, and
the various properties of the impulses that resulted were analyzed by our laboratory computer.

In Fig. 15 are the average values of the velocity, computed at the moment
that the impulse was completed (i.e., when the force trace crossed the zero-force
baseline) as a function of the size of the impulse (measured as the area under the
force-time curve). The relationship was strongly linear and seemed largely independent of the amplitude that the subject was required to make. This relationship would certainly not be surprising to a physicist, but it is perhaps comforting
that impulses in these movement situations follow Newtonian principles.

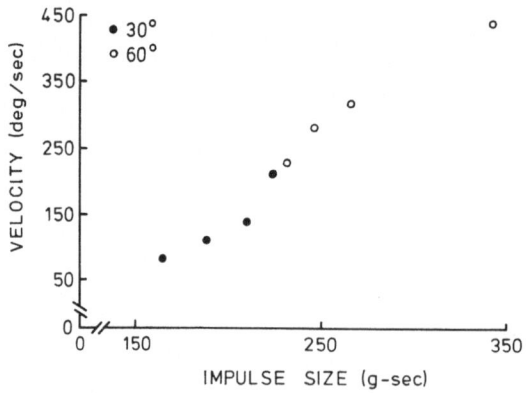

Fig. 15. The relationship between the velocity of a limb movement at the moment the impulse has stopped acting and the size of the impulse. (From Sherwood 1983)

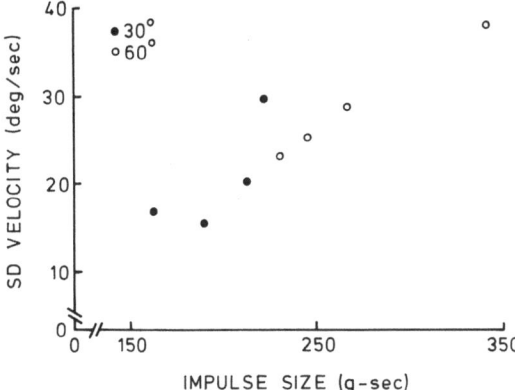

Fig. 16. The average within-subject SD of the velocity at the moment the impulse has stopped acting as a function of the impulse size. (From Sherwood 1983)

Variability in Velocity and Impulse Size

Important in our theorizing was the idea that the SD of the final velocity (i.e., at the moment the impulse has stopped acting) should be linearly related to the impulse size. Using the same motor responses just described, Sherwood (1983, 1984) also computed the within-subject SD of the velocity at the moment that the impulse had been terminated and plotted it against the size of the impulse as manipulated by the A and MT conditions. The relationship between SD (velocity) and impulse size, as shown in Fig. 16, is strongly linear, particularly so for the longer movement distance of 60° where the impulses were larger and more well defined. But, generally, there appeared to be a reasonably good fit of the data to the expectation that the variability in velocity should be related to impulse size.

Variability in Velocity and Average Velocity

A fundamental prediction, from Equation 6 above, is that the variability in the velocity achieved at the end of the agonist impulse should be directly related to the average velocity of the movement, calculated as the goal distance moved (A) divided by the goal MT (e.g., 60° in 150 ms or 400°/s). This relationship is plotted in Fig. 17 based on the four MT and two A conditions in Sherwood's ballistic-timing study. The average velocity of the responses (A/MT) was strongly linearly related to the SD of the velocity computed at the point where the impulse was terminated. The model again appears to predict this kind of relationship quite well. This is an important finding, as a major goal of the impulse-variability model was to relate simple descriptive features of a movement (e.g., its A and MT) to variabilities in certain kinematic features of the trajectories.

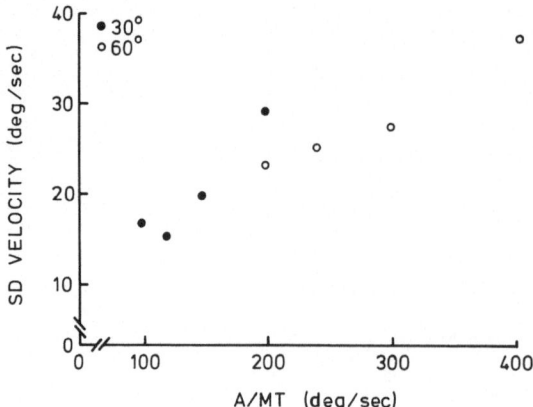

Fig. 17. The average within-subject SD of the velocity at the moment the impulse has stopped acting as a function of the average velocity of the response, A/MT. (From Sherwood 1983)

Summary

The findings above provide support for some of the fundamental assumptions of the impulse-variability model. In these simple tasks, at least, velocity and the variability in velocity are strongly related to impulse size; and variability in impulse size, in turn, is strongly related to the average velocity, A/MT. That variability in velocity is related to, and probably even determined by, the average velocity of the agonistic portion of the limb's trajectory, gives us strong encouragement to search further for fundamental relationships between certain measures of movement outcome, whose variability (or errors) can be related causally to the variability in the instructed velocity, or A/MT. We turn next to a number of such outcomes.

Various Predictions from the Model

Movement Time and Timing Error

One interesting finding to emerge from the 1960s and 1970s (e.g., Newell 1980; Newell, Hoshizaki, Carlton, and Halbert 1979; Newell, Carlton, and Halbert 1980; Schmidt 1969, 1982) was generated in ballistic-timing tasks. Here, error – scored as the SD of the MTs about the subject's own mean MT when attempting to produce a goal MT of, say, 150 ms – was positively related to the goal MT. In what some (e.g., Newell 1980; Schmidt 1982) have discussed in terms of "violations of the speed-accuracy trade-off effect," the finding is not that increases in speed (i.e., shorter MTs) lead to increased timing errors, but rather to the reverse: increased speed leads to *decreased* variable error in timing (VE_t). At first

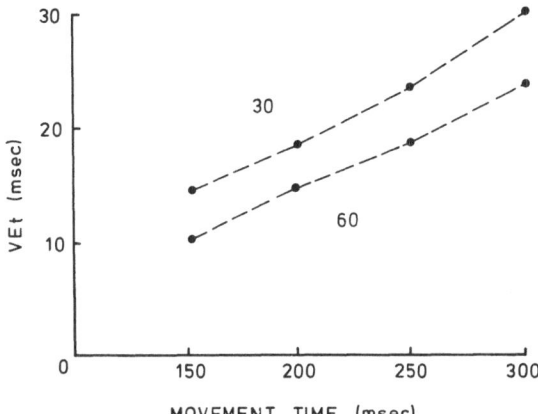

Fig. 18. Variable timing error (VE_t) in ballistic timing as a function of A and MT. (From Sherwood 1983)

glance, this phenomenon seems quite odd, but a closer examination reveals that it is predictable from the two impulse-variability models.

The impulse-variability models predict that VE_t from a ballistic timing task, or any task that has accuracy measured in terms of time, will be directly proportional to the goal MT. The details of the proofs will not be provided here, but they are in the original articles. Again, some of Sherwood's (1983) data support this prediction well. The task was ballistic timing and the A and MT were varied as described previously. VE_t was measured as the SD of the MTs actually produced, when the goal MTs were 150, 200, 250, or 300 ms. The plot of the VE_t against MT is shown in Fig. 18. It can be seen that the relationship between VE_t and MT is strongly linear for both A conditions, providing nice support for the model.

Velocity Effects

While the data within a given A condition provide strong support, the contrast across A conditions provides some difficulties. The model predicts that VE_t should be independent of A; yet there was a clear tendency for the shorter A conditions to produce larger VE_t. This effect of A on VE_t, even when the MT is held constant, implies that the *velocity* of the movement has an effect on VE_t over and above any simultaneous effects of MT. These so-called *velocity effects* were first shown by Newell et al. (1979, 1980), and his group has provided by far the most systematic study of them.

An example from some of their work is shown in Fig. 19, in which the VE_t divided by the MT is plotted against the average velocity of the movement (A/MT). The VE_t is divided by MT here in an attempt to "divide out" the effects of

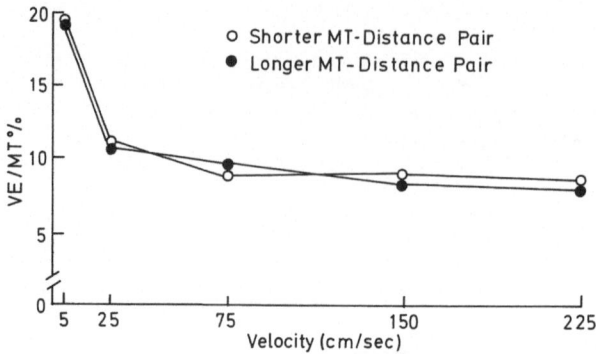

Fig. 19. Relative timing error expressed as $VE/MT\%$ in a ballistic timing task as a function of the average velocity. (From Newell et al. 1980)

MT on VE_t, as these two values are nearly proportional. After the MT effects are controlled in this way, any remaining effect of A or MT on VE_t/MT should be related to velocity, per se, uncontaminated by variations in MT. The figure shows that, as velocity increased, there was at first a sharp decline in timing error, followed by a more gradual decline as movement velocity was increased further. (See also Schmidt 1982, for a further discussion.)

These velocity effects can also be seen in a somewhat different way. In the two previous examples (Figs. 18, 19), the effect in these ballistic timing tasks was seen as an increase in the *timing* error (i.e., VE_t) as the amplitude (A) of the movement was decreased, with MT being held constant. But, one can also measure velocity effects as they influence *spatial* errors – measured as the SD of the movement's location at the moment the goal MT elapses ("W_e") – with the goal A held constant. Both the Schmidt et al. and Meyer et al. models predict (see their respective appendices for proofs) that, in ballistic-timing tasks with A constant, changes in MT (and, hence, velocity) should have no effect on the spatial errors. Yet, data from Sherwood (1983) contradict this prediction. As seen in Fig. 20, when the MT was increased, spatial errors (measured as "W_e" as described above) showed small (yet significant) decreases at each of the two values of A studied. Schmidt et al. (1979, Figure 13) in ballistic-timing tasks, and in reciprocal movements (Schmidt et al. 1979, Figure 17), have also shown these trends, but they were not statistically reliable in the earlier studies. In all of these cases, however, the velocity effect is opposite in direction to that found in experiments where A is manipulated with MT fixed (i.e., in Fig. 18, 19): decreased velocity (increased MT) leads to decreases (not increases) in error.

Neither the Schmidt et al. (1979) nor the Meyer et al. (1982) models can explain these velocity effects.[5] Both models predict that the velocity effect should

---

[5] We have not been able to complete a proof of no velocity effects from the Meyer et al. model as applied to the situation where VE_t is the dependent measure, but we suspect that it could be done. But proofs for the other three cases are in the respective papers.

be zero in such movement situations, and yet a considerable body of data now shows that such velocity effects are commonly found. Something is clearly wrong with our models in this respect.

How should the models be modified so that these effects can be predicted, while still retaining the effective predictions shown in the earlier parts of this section? We are not certain, but two possible suggestions are being considered at present. One of these, outlined by Sherwood and Schmidt (1980), and Sherwood (1983, 1984), is that A effects on VE_t (MT constant) are produced because there is a generally small, positive intercept in the relationship between force and force variability, whereas the models assume a zero intercept. This amounts to a situation in which movements with very low velocities (and hence low forces) have force variabilities that are far larger than predicted by the model. This error in predicting the amount of force variability becomes smaller as the movement velocity (and force) increases, because force and force variability are related more nearly proportionally as force increases. Thus velocity effects on VE_t are particularly large when velocity is low and become smaller as velocity increases – just what the data from Newell et al. (Fig. 19) show. We are encouraged by the possibility that by simply adding the additional assumption that force and force variability are related with a small positive intercept, our existing model (so modified) can explain the velocity effects.

A second possibility is related to the failure of our model to consider that force and time variability are correlated slightly negatively, with the size of the correlation increasing (in the negative direction) as the impulse size increases. Sherwood (1983, 1984) has argued that, if the correlation between force and time increases with impulse size, then a curvilinear relationship between the variability in velocity and A/MT results (contrary to Equation 6) and that this relationship should produce something like the velocity effects found. Whether or not this ef-

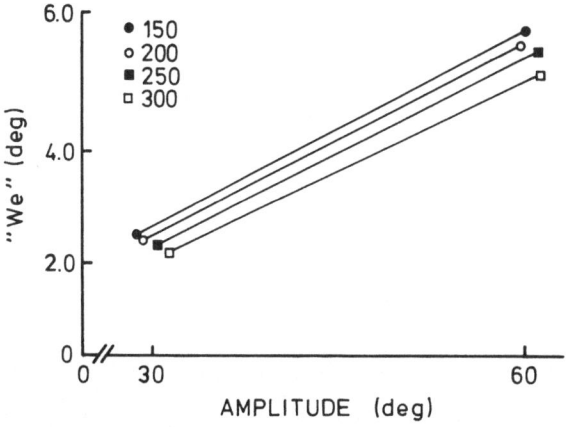

Fig. 20. The relationship between spatial errors (the SDs of the movement positions at the time the goal MT elapsed) and the amplitude and instructed MT in ballistic timing. (From Sherwood 1983)

fect is powerful enough to generate the rather large effects seen in Fig. 19 is unclear at present.

On the other hand, the velocity effects seen as changes in the spatial errors when MT is manipulated (with A fixed, as in Fig. 20) are considerably more difficult to understand. The problem is that modifications to the model as suggested in the previous paragraphs would seem to work here to make the discrepancies between the predicted and obtained velocity effects larger, not smaller. Thus, these velocity effects on spatial errors might represent yet another instance where the impulse-variability models have been inadequate in accounting for the effects of MT in simple tasks, as pointed out in various other places in this chapter. Additional future efforts need to be directed at this set of issues.

Movements with Large Force Requirements

We have mentioned earlier the issue about the form of the force-variability/force relationship being slightly nonlinear, contrary to the idealization we have used that force and force variability are proportional. We also mentioned the findings by Schmidt and Sherwood (1980), and to some extent Newell et al. (1982), that there may even be an inverted-U relationship between these variables, so that as force is increased beyond about 65% of the subject's maximum, decreases in force variability – not the expected increases – would be found. We now turn to an examination of the implications of these findings for movement behavior.

One obvious situation where these inverted-U phenomena could be relevant is in ballistic, preprogrammed actions where the force requirements are very large, such as might be involved in throwing, kicking, and punching actions so often found in various sport situations. We (Schmidt and Sherwood 1982) considered a laboratory version of one such task and asked whether variations in spatial accuracy in this rather "violent" response as a function of certain movement variables (e.g., the load to be moved and MT) could be predicted by the impulse-variability model, but with the addition of an inverted-U relationship between force and force variability.

Consider the simple model shown in Fig. 21, where a limb is being propelled to hit a stationary target. The plane of motion is horizontal, and the accuracy of target contact is measured in the *vertical* plane, much as it is when attempting to hit a ball with a bat in the game of baseball. If we imagine that there are sets of muscles acting on the limb at various angles to the resultant action, then we can have a basis for predicting the accuracy of these actions in the vertical (spatial) dimension as a function of the force requirements exerted in the horizontal dimension.

For example, if beginning with low force requirements, one experimentally increases the force by having the subjects move a progressively heavier object in a constant MT (in separate conditions), the force variability should increase with increased force, thereby causing increased variability in the trajectory and hence increased error. But, as the force requirements are increased further, beyond ap-

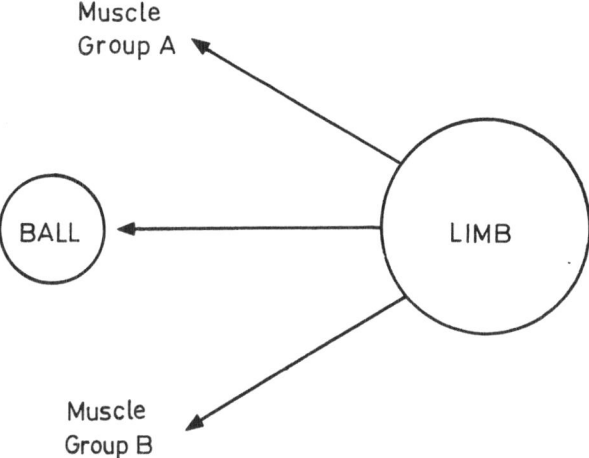

Fig. 21. A simple model for a limb being driven to a target by the contraction of two muscle groups. (From Schmidt and Sherwood 1982)

proximately 65% of the subjects' maximum (Fig. 9), the force variability should decrease, and one should observe a *decrease* in the spatial errors beyond this point. By the same argument, reducing *MT* so that the force requirements are increased beyond 65% of maximum should also reduce errors. These predictions do not seem to agree with common-sense expectations of the effects of these movement variables on accuracy.

Effects of mass. Our first experiment asked subjects to aim the extended right arm from a starting position to (and through) a target suspended on a cable. The movement was in the horizontal plane, the starting position had the arm pointing to the right, and the target was located in front of the shoulder. *MT* was controlled at 150 ms, and we added mass in various amounts (in separate experimental conditions) to a small handle the subject grasped. We also were able to estimate the percentage of maximal torque involved in these various conditions by using some simple assumptions and methods from biomechanics.

Errors in the vertical spatial dimension, expressed as variable error (*VE*, about the subject's own mean error) or total variability (*E*, about the target point), were computed across groups of trials for each experimental condition and are plotted in Fig. 22 as a function of the amount of mass added to the handle. As the force requirements were increased, there was an increase in error, but only to about 60–70% of maximum torque. Thereafter, increasing the mass on the handle caused the errors to *decrease,* so that the condition with the largest load (resulting in 89% of maximum torque) produced errors nearly equal to those found in the condition with the handle unloaded. Further, it is interesting that the point of maximum error was associated with about 60% of maximum torque, which is in good agreement with the point of maximum force variability found in our earlier experiments with static contractions (see Fig. 9).

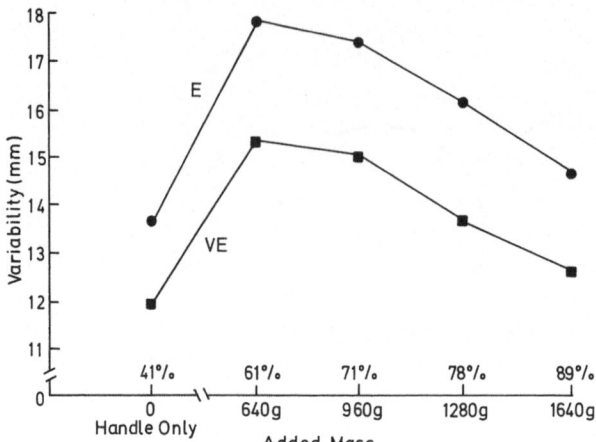

Fig. 22. Mean vertical spatial error expressed as *VE* and *E* in a rapid horizontal arm-swing task as a function of the inertial load applied to the handle. (From Schmidt and Sherwood 1982)

Effect of MT. In the same paper, we reported another experiment in which the force requirements were increased by decreasing *MT* under a constant load. The results of this study are shown in Fig. 23. As the *MT*s decreased, there was a gradual increase in the spatial accuracy to about 100 ms (or 50% of maximum torque). But decreasing *MT* further to 80 ms (where 84% of maximum torque was used, on average) resulted in a *decrease* in spatial movement error. Again, we are impressed by the finding that the point of maximum error (around 50% of maximum torque in these data) seems to agree with our estimates of maximum force variability seen in the static contractions.

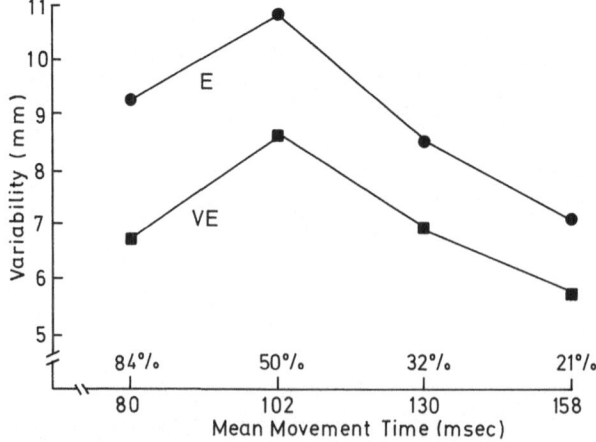

Fig. 23. Mean vertical spatial error expressed as *VE* and *E* in a rapid horizontal arm-swing task as a function of the instructed *MT*. (From Schmidt and Sherwood 1982)

Implications of inverted-U effects. These findings have a number of implications. First, from a theoretical viewpoint, the fact that force variability peaks and then decreases as the force increases further is contrary to both impulse-variability models' assumptions and will clearly make the predictions incorrect for any tasks with high force requirements. One possibility is to impose a boundary condition for the theories at about 65% of maximum torque, effectively limiting the range of movement possibilities to which the models are applicable. But a second, and preferable, solution is to create new models with these inverted-U relations between force and force variability included, so that the mathematics begins to subtract force variability when the forces are very large. Hopefully, then, such new models could account for some of the inverted-U relations found in movement tasks such as seen in Figs. 22 and 23.

But there are practical implications as well. First, it may be the case that this represents yet another situation where the speed-accuracy trade-off effect does not hold, and this information could perhaps be of use in instructing players in activities such as baseball where quick violent actions are required. We are often taught to "make contact" with the ball in these situations; translated, this means to swing easily and comfortably, certainly not as hard as possible. But, our data suggest that, in such situations, it may be reasonable to swing very hard, as spatial errors are apparently minimized in this way because of the force-variability principles. There are other advantages as well, such as increased timing accuracy, increased time to view a pitched ball before starting the swing, and a larger impact if the ball is contacted (see Schmidt 1982, for a discussion).

We should be cautious with these kinds of conclusions for a number of reasons. First, the movement studied in the Schmidt-Sherwood (1982) experiment is of the simplest kind, in which the limb must only be "thrown" through a target, with little or no control being exerted along the way. There is no requirement to stop the limb accurately in space or at a particular time, to make it coincide temporally with some external object (such as a *moving* ball), or to coordinate other limbs with it. Indeed, the movement was chosen *because* it was so simple and because the inverted-U, if present at all, seemed most likely to be uncovered in such a response. It could well be that, in more complicated tasks, the inverted-U relationship between error and force requirements will not hold.

In fact, another set of our data (Schmidt et al. 1985b), using a somewhat more complicated task, is contrary to this inverted-U expectation. We used a reversal task, in which the subject moved a lever via elbow flexion to a target 45° away, then reversed to move back through the starting position so that the time from the initial movement until the subject passed the starting position again achieved some goal MT value. We manipulated MT at seven different levels, with the smallest MT being associated with an essentially maximum-speed movement. The SDs of the movement reversal points (expressed as W_e) are given in Fig. 24 as a function of the time to the reversal point (essentially one-half the MT goal). Contrary to the findings in Fig. 23, as the MT decreased toward the subject's minimum, spatial error increased continuously, with the rate of error increase becoming especially large as the time to the reversal point became small. It would

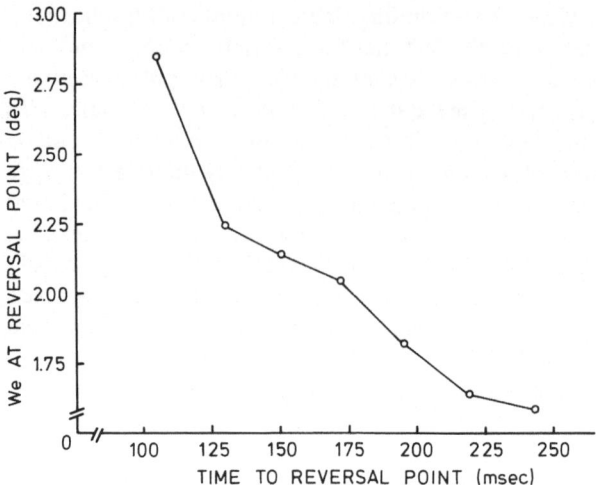

Fig. 24. Average within-subject SDs of the reversal point in a reversal task as a function of the instructed time to reversal. (From Schmidt et al. 1985 b)

appear that the addition of the requirement that the movement have a precisely timed and spatially accurate reversal point was sufficient to eliminate the inverted-U effect found in the simpler task. These results with reversal movements suggest that there is good reason to doubt the generality of the inverted-U effect, especially when the movements are complicated.

Problems in the Single-Aiming Paradigm

To this point, we have discussed only briefly the modeling and evidence concerning one of the most important paradigms at which both models are mainly directed – the single-aiming paradigm. Here, the subject makes a single movement of a hand-held stylus toward a target a few decimeters away, so that the *MT* is close to some goal *MT* (e.g., 150–250 ms). This response seems to obey the speed-accuracy principles rather well, as both *A* and *MT* have clear effects on error (see Fig. 1, for example). It is understandable that most attention has been directed towards this paradigm, as it is a modification of the Fitts (1954) task, which had been taken as the nearly classic paradigm for demonstrating speed-accuracy effects. So our attempts to model these phenomena in a different way have attracted some attention and criticism.

We have avoided discussing this paradigm until now primarily in the interest of clarity. With respect to the paradigms discussed so far in the chapter, there have been no serious objections from Meyer et al. or others about the assumptions we have made or the ways in which the tasks have been modeled. (But see the earlier section, Criticism of our Modeling Procedures, for minor exceptions.) Indeed, Meyer et al. have adopted most of our assumptions in generating their new model. But there are problems in modeling for the single-aiming paradigm, and it seemed clearer to treat these particular issues separately here.

Characteristics of Single-Aiming Tasks

Why should a particular paradigm, one of many that show speed-accuracy effects, be singled out for special treatment? We are not certain that it is wise to do so, but it does present some rather different features as compared with the other tasks that have been discussed so far. In particular, single-aiming tasks are three-dimensional, involving clearly more than movement in a single dimension or plane as the other tasks do. More importantly, we recognized long ago (Schmidt et al. 1978) that the movement's endpoint (upon which measures of error are based) is determined not only by movement in the horizontal dimension (which the models treat), but also by movements in the vertical dimension (which the models do not treat). Specifically, *where* the stylus lands is determined in part by *when* the stylus is brought down to the plane of the target, much as where an airplane lands on the runway will be dependent on when the pilot touches it down. Another problem is that a portion of the deceleration for the limb is provided (both in the horizontal and vertical planes) by impact with the target area, so that not all of the speed-accuracy effect can be clearly related to the variability in the actions of the relevant muscles; and the amount of force on the target is directly related to A and inversely related to MT (Teasdale and Schmidt, 1985). All of these factors together have made the paradigm rather "special," at least for us, providing considerable difficulties in modeling.

Our Single-Aiming Model Criticized

Meyer et al. (1982), who generally accepted our modeling in various movement paradigms, criticized our treatment of the single-aiming paradigm. They pointed out that, rather than predicting that W_e in aiming should be proportional to A/MT as we claimed, our model really predicts that W_e should be proportional to A, and essentially independent of MT. They are correct in their criticism, in our view, and we cannot argue with their conclusions. Of course, from Fig. 1 and other data, we know that MT has powerful effects on W_e in this task; thus our model, applied to this paradigm, is not only logically incorrect but does not predict the empirical facts.

Physical laws. Meyer et al. argued that we misapplied physical principles in coming to our conclusion that W_e in aiming should be proportional to A/MT. Perhaps it amounts to "splitting hairs," but the error arose in a quite different way than they imply, and thus we are not really as ignorant about Newtonian principles as Meyer et al. portray us to be. We recognized fairly early (Schmidt et al. 1978) that our model, considered in the horizontal plane only, predicts that W_e is independent of MT – a clear difficulty. In an attempt to solve this problem, we reasoned as follows. We had assumed (correctly, we think) that the variability in the velocity of the stylus at about the movement midpoint was proportional to A/MT (see Equation 6 in the present chapter). And, since the stylus was traveling horizontally as it was dropping vertically near the target, variability in horizontal velocity would be translated into variability in where the stylus landed. Therefore, we reasoned (incorrectly, we now realize) that the variability in where the stylus landed (W_e) should also be proportional to A/MT. Thus the reasoning that led to the erroneous prediction that $W_e \propto A/MT$ resulted from an additional assumption about how the stylus "landed" on the target surface, and *not* because we used Newtonian kinematic principles incorrectly. While our earlier reasoning might appear correct, it ignored the fact that the variability in the time to drop is not constant, but rather is proportional to MT. When this feature of the movement is considered, the model actually predicts that W_e should be independent of MT, an unacceptable result.

Movement dynamics oversimplified. Our modeling of the single-aiming task was also criticized by Meyer et al. (1982, p. 457) for considering only the accelerative aspects of the movement to the neglect of deceleration. As we have just discussed, and contrary to Meyer et al.'s statements, we were very concerned with the dynamics of the action as the limb approached the target area, although we did not model this feature of the movement formally. We did, however, deal with the decelerative aspects formally for our one-dimensional reciprocal paradigm (Schmidt et al., 1979, p. 451). Also, we did not say, as Meyer et al. claimed (on p. 454) that the movement acts in "free fall" during deceleration; to the contrary, this aspect of the movement was considered to be controlled by the same motor program that controls acceleration, and thus to be subject to the same sources of variability. Finally, we find it curious that Meyer et al. would criticize our model for oversimplifying the movement dynamics at the end of the aiming response and then propose a model which itself considers only the horizontal aspects of the action; indeed, all of the complicated features of aiming movements, discussed above, are ignored in their modeling of them, as they freely admit. In retrospect, it seems clear that both models are inadequate with respect to the movement dynamics involved in aiming movements, and that considerable modeling improvements will be made by considering these features.

Other Modeling Difficulties for Aiming Tasks

In addition to the above criticisms of our modeling of aiming tasks, there are other difficulties that apply to both the Schmidt et al. and Meyer et al. attempts. These are summarized in the next few sections.

Acceleration-time functions. Meyer et al. derived a specific form of the acceleration-time function which allows $W_e \propto A/MT$. In fact, their modeling is very interesting and elegant in this regard, as they *begin* with the empirical relationship that $W_e \propto A/MT$ and then derive the mathematical acceleration-time function that produces it. One feature of these functions is their mirror-image symmetry, so that the accelerative and decelerative impulses, after one of them is inverted and reversed, would be congruent. We have presented evidence here (Zelaznik and Schmidt 1983) that this symmetry assumption does not hold in aiming (see Fig. 12), with the impulse for acceleration having a considerably longer duration and smaller peak amplitude than the impulse for deceleration. Also, Meyer et al. provided none of their own (or others') evidence that actual force-time curves had the mathematical form that they require, although various aspects of their curve forms do appear roughly realistic to us. Also, probably associated with these asymmetries, we find that the spatial trajectories of the movements are not symmetrical, with a gradual rise in the hand to a point considerably past the movement midpoint, and then a rather abrupt drop toward the target. And, this peak in amplitude appears to shift toward the target slightly as the MT decreases (Zelaznik and Schmidt 1983).

Force-time rescalability and shape constancy. A second critical assumption of both models, as mentioned previously, is that of shape constancy as the acceleration-time curves are increased or decreased in amplitude and/or extended or short-ened in duration. As we discussed in a previous section, there is good reason to suspect that this assumption may hold for many of the tasks that we have stud-ied, but it is clear from two investigations (Schmidt et al., 1985 a; Zelaznik and Schmidt 1983) that it does *not* hold for aiming tasks. (This is yet another reason why aiming tasks seem "special" to us.) On the contrary, the time from the be-ginning of the movement to peak acceleration and the time from peak decelera-tion to the end of the movement are essentially constant and are not proportional to MT as this assumption requires. (Review Figs. 12 and 13 and related discussion about this point.) The evidence suggests that this critical assumption, on which both models are based, may be incorrect for aiming movements. It appears that our understanding of how impulses vary when A and/or MT are manipulated is incomplete or incorrect, suggesting that modifications to generalized motor pro-gram theory – at least for aiming movements – are needed.

Impulse Variability and Aiming: A Summary

It is ironic that the largest failure of the impulse-variability models to date is with respect to the movements that originally motivated the models – aiming tasks. Both models fail to consider the reasonably complex three-dimensional nature of these movements, such as the observations (a) that the target surface provides considerable deceleration for the limb, (b) that the variability in time to drop and in other temporal aspects of the vertical trajectory are probably nearly pro-portional to MT, and (c) that where the limb lands depends on when it lands.

Also, both models have apparently made false assumptions about the nature of the changes in the acceleration-time curves with changes in A and MT. There are many smaller problems as well, such as the nonlinearities and nonzero intercepts in the force-variability/force relationship. It seems clear to us that neither of the impulse-variability models is capable of accounting for the critical facts about aiming tasks.

Problems with Simple, Uniplanar Responses

In contrast to the serious difficulties the impulse variability models have had with three-dimensional single-aiming responses, we had been encouraged that the empirical facts were reasonably well handled by the model for the single-joint uniplanar responses discussed earlier in this chapter. In the uniplanar responses (e.g., ballistic timing, reciprocal tasks, and reversal tasks), a few troublesome deviations from the predicted results have emerged (e.g., velocity effects), and we thought that these could be handled by small adjustments to the form of the force-variability/force functions. But recently we have found more serious difficulties in these paradigms that seem to require more serious changes in the model even for these situations.

In the reversal task, where the subject must make a single reversal in direction to achieve a given MT, our model predicts that spatial variability (W_e) in the reversal point should be independent of the MT and proportional to A. Results like these have been produced previously in reciprocal tasks, which we considered to be a series of reversal tasks "strung together" (e.g., Schmidt et al. 1979, Fig. 17). But in a careful examination of these effects in reversal tasks recently, Schmidt et al. (1985b) have found a number of contradictions to these expectations. While increases in A with a constant MT produced nearly linear increases in W_e as we expected, the effect of MT with a constant A showed a large MT-W_e trade-off. These data were discussed previously in another context (Fig. 24) and they reveal that decreases in MT produce increases in W_e, particularly when the MTs are short. These results, in addition to some other unpublished findings, lead us to the view that, while our model predicts the effects of A reasonably well, it is not effective in predicting the effects of MT. This MT effect with reversal tasks, more than anything else, has led us to abandon our impulse-variability model even for these uniplanar responses for which early success could be claimed.

General Discussion

Effectiveness of the Impulse-Variability Models

The success of impulse-variability models to explain speed-accuracy relationships in rapid motor tasks must perhaps be viewed from two different perspectives. In terms of the first viewpoint, from which these models have been very successful, the impulse-variability models have provided a plausible alternative hypothesis to the earlier position that speed-accuracy relationships were determined mainly by feedback processes. Our model (Schmidt et al. 1979) and later Meyer et al.'s (1982) version both emphasized that impulse variability was probably an important contributor to these speed-accuracy relationships and that it may even provide a complete explanation when the movements are very rapid and feedback cannot be used to any important extent. Exactly how these impulse-variability processes should be modeled is certainly open to question, but the viewpoint that variability in motor-output processes is responsible for errors in rapid movements has received a great deal of support, and it might even be said that this overall position is reasonably well accepted by today's researchers in motor control.

But from the second viewpoint, where both (a) the assumptions and modeling methods and (b) the accuracy of predicting the empirical facts are considered, the impulse-variability models can be shown to be rather seriously lacking. These aspects are summarized briefly below.

Assumptions and Modeling Methods

Certainly, two of the major assumptions of both impulse-variability models appear incorrect, and others have had some doubts raised about them. Probably most important is the finding that, in aiming responses at least, impulses do not behave as we have assumed when the A and MT are changed experimentally. We and Meyer et al. had assumed that impulses contract and expand along both the force and time dimensions while retaining the basic mathematical form (force and time rescalability, in Meyer et al.'s terms). But to the contrary, impulses in aiming responses appear to have a constant interval from the beginning of the movement until peak acceleration, and a constant interval from the peak deceleration until the end of the movement. Also, contrary to the Meyer et al. (1982) model (but not the Schmidt et al. model), the impulses are not symmetrical in form, and the movement trajectory is not symmetrical either. On the other hand, the assumed changes in impulses with A and MT do appear to hold at least roughly for a number of other classes of movement, mainly involving uniplanar, single-joint actions (Schmidt, in press). Why the variations in the form of the impulses appear to be different for these different paradigms is certainly not clear, but our efforts to understand single-aiming responses with this particular assumption will almost certainly be inadequate.

A second assumption deals with the basic form of the force-variability/force function. Most agree that force variability generally rises with force requirements. But there has been debate about whether or not this function is linear and, if it is, whether or not force variability is proportional to force as impulse-variability models have assumed. And, there is some evidence that the function has an inverted-U form (Sherwood and Schmidt 1980). After reviewing the evidence, we have come to accept Newell et al.'s (in press) position that force variability is a negatively accelerating positive function of force and that inverted-U phenomena are probably a result of failures to control adequately the time to peak force. When such times to peak force are controlled (e.g., Sherwood et al. 1985), inverted-U functions have not been found in our reversal tasks as a function of MT. So, conceptualizing the force-variability/force relationship as a proportional one has probably led to at least some of the problems in prediction. In addition, the assumption (by Schmidt et al. 1979, only) that the variations in impulse amplitude and impulse duration are independent is generally not correct.

Predicting the Empirical Facts

At a coarse level, some of the important empirical relationships found in various experiments appear to be reasonably well predicted by the impulse-variability models. Increasing A (MT constant) in ballistic timing, in reversal and reciprocal tasks, and in single-aiming generally leads to major increases in spatial errors and only minor changes in measures of temporal error. Also, in ballistic timing, increasing MT (A fixed) generally leads to increases in timing errors and only small effects on spatial errors. On the other hand, the small, but systematic, velocity effects probably cannot be predicted by either model.

More serious for the Schmidt et al. model are the predicted effects of MT. The model is clearly inadequate in this regard for single-aiming movements, as Meyer et al. have pointed out. But in some of the other paradigms we have studied (e.g., the reversal task), we find increases in the spatial variability of the reversal points with decreased MT which are clearly contrary to the predicted independence between these two variables. We are not certain what Meyer et al. predict in the reversal task, as they do not address it as one of their target paradigms. But if their model does predict MT effects such as we have found empirically, it is possible that they may have found the proper solution, as the reversal paradigm is one in which the assumptions of force and time rescalability *do* appear to hold. But this still leaves the problem of their modeling in single-aiming responses, as force-time rescalability apparently does not hold here.

Some Possible Solutions and Future Directions

Both impulse-variability models, while perhaps conceptually reasonable with respect to the idea that speed-accuracy trade-offs are caused by variations in movement output rather than by limitations in feedback processing, seem inadequate with respect to the more detailed statements about how such variability occurs and how it leads to errors in movement. In the final section of this chapter, we provide some suggestions for future efforts to model these phenomena.

First of all, we must come to understand how impulses change as the variables of critical interest here (e.g., A, MT, mass to be moved) are varied experimentally. And, we must develop rules that apply to all the various paradigms, lest we have theories of speed-accuracy phenomena that are so paradigm-specific as to be nearly useless. Work on these questions is currently underway in our lab (e.g., Schmidt et al. 1985 a; Shapiro and Schmidt 1983; Shapiro and Walter 1985; Sherwood 1983) and in others' laboratories (e.g., Newell et al., 1982, in press; Soechting and Lacquanti 1983) to isolate the invariances in force-time functions as a wide variety of movement requirements are altered (e.g., movement direction, movement trajectory, as well as A and MT). Also, of course, we must be certain that Newell et al. (in press) are correct in their formulations about force-variability/force functions, and further work on how impulse-duration variability varies with MT is needed in various movement contexts. When these principles of movement control are better understood, modeling efforts using these newer ideas about invariances will probably be more successful in predicting the empirical facts.

But some other features of the neuromuscular situations will probably have to be added, as we can point to at least two important principles that have been ignored in previous modeling attempts. The first of these is the well-known force-velocity relationship, where the force that a muscle applies (with a given level of neurological activation) decreases as the velocity of shortening increases (Fenn and Marsh 1950; Wilkie 1950; see Partridge 1979, for a review). Such effects are often included in biomechanical models to provide the damping necessary to allow the model to predict the smooth achievement of target endpoints seen in skilled motor behavior. These muscle properties – especially when they deal with velocity, which is a major independent variable in impulse-variability models – seem particularly important to consider; yet they are currently absent.

A second feature that could be included in future modeling efforts is the tendency for muscle to behave like a "complicated spring." In particular, as the length of a muscle (again, under constant neurological activation) is increased, the tension produced (and presumably its variability) increases as well (e. g. Rack and Westbury 1969; see also Partridge 1979). This seems particularly important to consider in the rapid movement tasks used here, as the force (and variability) produced by a muscle will be dependent not only on the neurological activation but also on the length of the muscle at that moment. In reversal tasks, for example, variations in the force that flexes the elbow will lead to variations in the position of the limb at the time the antagonist muscle is activated, leading to additional variability during deceleration because of the length-tension relationship.

There is clearly much to be done before speed-accuracy effects in rapid movement situations can be understood. But we are encouraged that, with increased understanding of some fundamentals of impulse control and impulse variability, a direction seems provided that has a reasonable chance of predicting a wide variety of empirical phenomena.

Acknowledgments. R. A. Schmidt was supported by Grant No. BNS-80-23125 from the National Science Foundation, Memory and Cognitive Processes Program. We would like to express our appreciation to Herbert Heuer, Uwe Kleinbeck, David Meyer, Karl Newell, and Charles Wright for their many helpful comments on earlier drafts of this chapter.

References

Armstrong, T. R. (1970). *Training for the production of memorized movement patterns* (Technical Report No. 26). Ann Arbor: University of Michigan, Human Performance Center.

Carter, M. C., and Shapiro, D. C. (1984). Control of sequential movements: Evidence for generalized motor programs. *Journal of Neurophysiology, 52,* 787–796.

Crossman, E. R. F. W., and Goodeve, P. J. (1983). Feedback control of hand movements and Fitts' law. Proceedings of the Experimental Society, Oxford, 1963. *Quarterly Journal of Experimental Psychology, 35A,* 251–278.

Denier van der Gon, J. J., and Thuring, J. P. H. (1965). The guiding of human writing movements. *Kybernetik, 2,*145–148.

Fenn, W. O., and Marsh, B. S. (1950). Muscular force at different speeds of shortening. *Journal of Physiology* (London), *85,* 277–297.

Fitts, P. M. (1954). The information capacity of the human motor system in controlling the amplitude of movement. *Journal of Experimental Psychology, 47,* 381–391.

Fullerton, G. S., and Cattell, J. M. (1892). On the perception of small differences. *University of Pennsylvania Philosophical Series,* No. 2.

Ghez, C. (1979). Contributions of central programs to rapid limb movements in the cat. In H. Asanuma and V. J. Wilson (Eds.) *Integration in the nervous system.* Tokyo: Isaku-Shoin.

Ghez, C., and Vicario, D. (1978). The control of rapid limb movement in the cat: II. Scaling of isometric force adjustments. *Experimental Brain Research, 33,* 191–202.

Hollerbach, J. M. (1981). An oscillation theory of handwriting. *Biological Cybernetics, 39,* 139–156.

Howarth, C. I., Beggs, W. D. A., and Bowden, J. M. (1971). The relationship between speed and accuracy of movement aimed at a target. *Acta Psychologica, 35,* 207–218.

Jenkins, W. O. (1947). The discrimination and reproduction of motor adjustments with various tapes of aircraft controls. *American Journal of Psychology, 60,* 396–406.

Keele, S. W. (1968). Movement control in skilled motor performance. *Psychological Bulletin, 70,* 387–403.

Leikind, B. J. (1985). A generalization of constant acceleration formulas of Newtonian kinematics. Manuscript submitted for publication, UCLA.

Merton, P. A. (1974). The properties of the human muscle servo. *Brain Research, 71,* 475–478.

Meyer, D. E., Smith, J. E. K., and Wright, C. E. (1982). Models for the speed and accuracy of aimed movements. *Psychological Review, 89,* 449–482.

Michon, J. A. (1967). *Timing in temporal tracking.* Soesterberg, The Netherlands: Institute for Perception RNO-TNO.

Newell, K. M. (1980). The speed-accuracy paradox in movement control: errors of time and space. In G. E. Stelmach (Ed.), *Tutorials in motor behavior.* Amsterdam: North-Holland.

Newell, K. M., and Carlton, L. G. (1983). On the force and force variability relationship. *Bulletin of the Psychonomic Society, 21,* 336 (Abstract).

Newell, K. M., Carlton, L. G., and Carlton, M. J. (1982). The relationship of impulse to response timing error. *Journal of Motor Behavior, 1982, 14,* 24–45.

Newell, K. M., Carlton, L. G., Carlton, M. J., and Halbert, J. A. (1980). Velocity as a factor in movement timing accuracy. *Journal of Motor Behavior, 12,* 47–56.

Newell, K. M., Carlton, L. G., and Hancock, P. A. (in press). A kinetic analysis of response variability. *Psychological Bulletin.*

Newell, K. M., Hoshizaki, L. E. F., Carlton, M. J., and Halbert, J. A. (1979). Movement time and velocity as determinants of movement timing accuracy. *Journal of Motor Behavior, 11,* 49–58.

Noble, M. E., and Bahrick, H. P. (1956). Response generalization as a function of intratask response similarity. *Journal of Experimental Psychology, 51,* 405–412.

Partridge, L. D. (1979). Muscle properties: A problem for the motor physiologist. In R. E. Talbot and D. R. Humphrey (Eds.), *Posture and movement.* New York: Raven.

Pew, R. W. (1974). Human perceptual-motor performance. In B. H. Kantowitz (Ed.), *Human information processing: Tutorials in performance and cognition.* Hillsdale, NJ: Erlbaum.

Rack, P. M. H., and Westbury, D. R. (1969). The effects of length and stimulus rate on tension in the isometric cat soleus muscle. *Journal of Physiology, 204,* 443–460.

Raibert, M. H. (1977). *Motor control and learning by the state-space model* (Technical Report No. AI-TR-439). Cambridge: MIT, Artificial Intelligence Laboratory.

Schmidt, R. A. (1969). Movement time as a determiner of timing accuracy. *Journal of Experimental Psychology, 79,* 43–47.

Schmidt, R. A. (1975). A schema theory of discrete motor skill learning. *Psychological Review, 86,* 225–260.

Schmidt, R. A. (1976). Control processes in motor skills. *Exercise and Sport Sciences Reviews, 4,* 229–261.

Schmidt, R. A. (1982). Motor control and learning: A behavioral emphasis. Champaign, IL: Human Kinetics Press.

Schmidt, R. A. (in press). The search for invariance in skilled movement behavior. *Research Quarterly for Exercise and Sport.*

Schmidt, R. A., Gielen, C. C. A. M., and Zelaznik, H. N. (1985a). Sources of variability in single aiming responses: Contributions of the decelerative phase. Paper read at the NASPSPA annual meeting, Gulfport, MS, June, 1985.

Schmidt, R. A., and Sherwood, D. E. (1982). An inverted-U relation between spatial error and force requirements in rapid limb movements: Further evidence for the impulse-variability model. *Journal of Experimental Psychology: Human Perception and Performance, 8,* 158–170.

Schmidt, R. A., Zelaznik, H. N., and Frank, J. S. (1978). Sources of inaccuracy in rapid movement. In G. E. Stelmach (Ed.) *Information processing in motor control and learning.* New York: Academic Press.

Schmidt, R. A., Zelaznik, H. N., Hawkins, B., Frank, J. S., and Quinn, J. T. (1979). Motor-output variability: A theory for the accuracy of rapid motor acts. *Psychological Review, 86,* 415–451.

Schmidt, R. A., Sherwood, D. E., and Walter, C. B. Manuscript in preparation, UCLA, 1985b.

Shapiro, D. C. (1977). A preliminary attempt to determine the duration of a motor program. In D. M. Landers and R. W. Christina (Eds.), *Psychology of motor behavior and sport I.* Champaign, IL: Human Kinetics Press.

Shapiro, D. C., and Walter, C. B. The control of rapid positioning movements with spatiotemporal constraints. Manuscript submitted for publication, 1985.

Shapiro, D. C., and Schmidt, R. A. (1983). The control of direction in rapid aiming movements. *Society for Neuroscience Abstracts, 9* (2), 1031. (Abstract)

Sherwood, D. E. (1983). *The impulse-variability model: Tests of the major assumptions and predictions.* Ph. D. dissertation, University of Southern California, 1983.

Sherwood, D. E. Major assumptions and predictions of the impulse-variability model. Manuscript submitted for publication, UCLA, 1984.

Sherwood, D. E., and Schmidt, R. A. (1980). The relationship between force and force variability in minimal and near-maximal static and dynamic contractions. *Journal of Motor Behavior, 12,* 75–89.

Sherwood, D. E., Schmidt, R. A., and Walter, C. B. Manuscript in preparation, UCLA, 1984.

Soechting, J. F., and Lacquaniti, F. (1983). Modification of trajectory of a pointing movement in response to a change in target location. *Journal of Neurophysiology, 49,* 548–564.

Teasdale, N., and Schmidt, R. A. (1985). Horizontal impact in the deceleration process of single aiming movements. Paper presented at the NASPSPA annual meeting, Gulfport, MS, June, 1985.

Wilkie, D. R. (1950). The relation between force and velocity in human muscle. *Journal of Physiology* (London), *110,* 249–280.

Wing, A. M., and Kristofferson, A. B. (1973). The timing of interresponse intervals. *Perception and Psychophysics, 13,* 455–460.

Woodworth, R. S. (1901). On the voluntary control of the force of movement. *Psychological Review, 8,* 350–359.

Zelaznik, H. N., and Schmidt, R. A. (1983). Kinematic properties of single-aiming movements. *Bulletin of the Psychonomic Society, 21,* 335. (Abstract)

Appendix

In this appendix we show that the displacement of a particle subject to an acceleration that is a function of time will always be proportional to the acceleration and to the square of the time that the acceleration is applied as long as the form of the acceleration is preserved when the acceleration duration is changed. Further, if the acceleration function is symmetric, then replacing the acceleration with its average value will yield both the correct velocity and the correct displacement at the end of the acceleration.

Imagine an acceleration function that begins at time $-T/2$ and ends at time $T/2$ applied to a particle that begins at rest at $x = 0$. We will suppose that the initial position and velocity of the particle are zero. (The generalization to any initial conditions is easy and does not affect the results derived here.) The particle's displacement at $t = T/2$ is found by integrating the acceleration once to get the velocity as a function of time and then integrating again to find the position as a function of time. Thus the position at time $T/2$ is given by

$$x\left(\frac{T}{2}\right) = \int\limits_{-T/2}^{T/2} dt' \int\limits_{-T/2}^{t'} dt'' \, a\,(t''). \tag{A1}$$

This is a double integral over the variable t' and t''. The integration is carried out over the region of $t' - t''$ space above the line $t' = t''$, to the left of the line $t'' = -T/2$, and below the line $t'' = T/2$. We may integrate over t' first. Thus,

$$x\left(\frac{T}{2}\right) = \int\limits_{-T/2}^{T/2} dt'' \int\limits_{t''}^{T/2} dt' \, a\,(t''). \tag{A2}$$

Since $a\,(t'')$ is not a function of t' we may remove it from the t' integral,

$$x\left(\frac{T}{2}\right) = \int\limits_{-T/2}^{T/2} dt'' \, a\,(t'') \left(\frac{T}{2} - t''\right). \tag{A3}$$

Expanding the integral yields

$$x\left(\frac{T}{2}\right) = \frac{T}{2} \int_{-T/2}^{T/2} dt'' \, a(t'') - \int_{-T/2}^{T/2} dt'' \, a(t'') \, t''. \tag{A4}$$

The first integral on the right-hand side of Equation A4 is the average value of $a(t)$, and the second integral is proportional to the average value of $a(t)\,t$, or the first moment of $a(t)$. We define

$$A = \frac{1}{T} \int_{-T/2}^{T/2} dt \, a(t) \quad \text{and} \quad BT = -\frac{2}{T} \int_{-T/2}^{T/2} dt \, a(t) \, t. \tag{A5}$$

Then Equation A4 is

$$x\left(\frac{T}{2}\right) = \frac{1}{2}(A + B) \, T^2. \tag{A6}$$

Now, every function can be written as the sum of an even or symmetric part and an odd or antisymmetric part. That is,

$$a(t) = a_e(t) + a_0(t),$$

where

$$a_e(t) = (\tfrac{1}{2})[a(t) + a(-t)] \tag{A7}$$

and

$$a_0(t) = (\tfrac{1}{2})[a(t) - a(-t)].$$

Clearly any odd part of the acceleration will contribute nothing to A while any even part of the acceleration will contribute nothing to B.

We may now draw the following conclusions. From Equations A5 and A6 we see that the displacement of a particle subject to any acceleration is always proportional to the amplitude of the acceleration and to the square of the movement time. The form of the acceleration function must be preserved as the time T is varied for this to be true. Furthermore, if the acceleration function is symmetric, then the displacement of the particle at the time $T/2$ will be $x(T/2) = (\tfrac{1}{2})AT^2$. That is, by replacing the acceleration function with its average value we obtain the correct velocity, as is well known from the usual impulse theory, and we obtain the correct displacement as well.

The Control of Simple Movements by Multisensory Information

C. I. Howarth and W. D. A. Beggs

Contents

Introduction

Simple movements are those with a clear beginning and a clear end, with an economical progression between the two. They have been much studied because their accuracy and timing can be measured comparatively easily, and the relationship between movement time and accuracy is the commonest statistic to be used in testing theories of the control of movement. One hopes that an understanding of simple movements can be generalised to improve our understanding of complex movements, but simple movements are of practical as well as theoretical interest. Common acts such as kicking or throwing, picking up objects and putting them down, pointing or aiming are all simple movements.

Despite their simplicity, the study of such movements has become very confusing, with many different theories leading to many different experimental situations and many different kinds of measurement. Some of the resulting controversies have been a consequence of this. One of the purposes of this paper is to offer a classification of existing data and experimental situations in a way which makes it possible to map data on to theories in less ambiguous ways.

Our first step is to make a clear distinction between the several different ways in which movement performance can be measured. Measurements of constant and variable errors show very different effects of other variables such as movement time or distance. We will confine most of our discussion in this paper to measures of the dispersion of hits around a target, or variable errors. It is, however, important to consider the way in which these are measured. In a task where a stylus hits a target which is normal to the direction of movement, all variable errors can be thought of as errors of aiming (e.g. in the task described by

Howarth, Beggs, and Bowden 1971). Here, the errors were measured at right angles to the direction of motion of the hand.

In the classic Fitts' tapping task, however, where the target is on a table, errors may be errors of aiming or errors of stopping. In the latter case, errors are measured in the same direction as the movement of the hand. Figure 1 shows the difference between measures of aiming and measures of stopping.

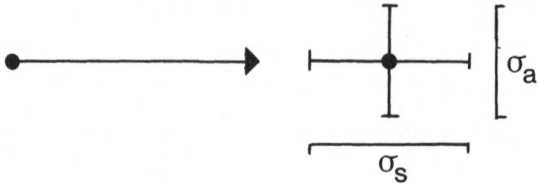

Fig. 1. Errors of aiming (σ_a) and errors of stopping (σ_s)

This is, of course, an oversimplification, because the trajectory of the subject's hand as it approaches the target may well change as a function of the precise parameters of the task or other factors. In practice, the difference between errors of aiming and errors of stopping may become blurred.

Nevertheless, we believe that it is important to make this theoretical distinction as an aid to gaining an understanding of the processes which may produce these different sorts of error, and to design experiments which examine performance in ways which can test theories about these processes. Unfortunately, some experimental paradigms, such as the one used by Fitts (1954) and his many followers, confuse errors of aiming with errors of stopping, and constant errors with variable errors. As a result, the data yielded by such paradigms are almost useless in evaluating modern theories of motor control.

Experiments on speed-accuracy trade-off may be either paced or unpaced. In paced experiments the accuracy of timing, as well as of movement, may be measured, but the dependent variable is usually positional accuracy. In unpaced experiments, the dependent variable is usually movement time, with the subject being asked to move as quickly as possible to targets of varying sizes. The positional accuracy may still be measured, but usually only as an error or failure to hit the target. The accuracy achieved within a target is seldom measured (but see Bainbridge and Sanders 1972). Paced and unpaced experiments often give similar results, but there are characteristic differences which will be discussed later.

It is also important to distinguish between movements which are under sensory control (closed loop) and those which are not (open loop). Many theories of movement control have stressed that a movement may be partly open-loop during its execution, either because there is not enough time to exercise control (Howarth et al. 1971; Keele 1968) or because the subject choses not to use the available information (Zelaznik, Shapiro, and McColsky 1981).

Our theory of the control of simple movements first described by Howarth et al. (1971) is concerned with the relationship between movement time and variable errors of aiming. The second purpose of this paper is to present an up-to-date account of our theory and to try to relate it to other work. We will make no attempt to account for constant errors or errors of stopping, on the grounds that rather different mechanisms are involved in determining such measures. Most of the experiments to be considered will involve paced movements.

The theory is concerned with the control of movement by sensory information and assumes that the accuracy of movement, as measured by the variable error of aiming, is determined by only two factors: (1) The accuracy of the sensory information available and (2) the time available to respond to this information.

Other models of motor performance, generally those whose focus of interest is very rapid movements, have made very different assumptions. For example, Klapp (1975) and Schmidt, Zelaznik, Hawkins, Frank and Quinn (1979) have assumed that motor, rather than perceptual, factors are crucial. The interesting work of Bizzi, Polit and Morasso (1976) and Kelso (1977) suggests that limbs can be moved to positions relative to the body simply on the basis of muscle coding of these target locations. These approaches are very different from our own and describe very different situations. As Keele (1981) points out, these different ways of thinking about motor performance may be complementary, and explain different phases of movement towards a target.

Intersensory Localisation

The sensory information which is potentially available to control limb movements comes from many sources. It may be reafferent information derived from the monitoring of motor output, it may be kinaesthetic information from senses in the muscles and joints, or it may be visual if we happen to be looking at the limb, or at the target towards which it is moving. Our fundamental assumption is that the accuracy of movement primarily depends on the accuracy with which we know the relationship between the present position of a limb and its final or target position (Howarth 1978), although other models, such as the mass-spring model, do not make this assumption.

Judgements of the relative positions of objects are called intersensory localisations when the objects are perceived by different senses. A typical intersensory localisation experiment is one in which the subject sits in a dark room in which a single spot of light appears. At the same time he touches a spot at arm's length in front of him, which he cannot see. He is then asked to judge whether the spot of light is to the left or to the right of the touched spot.

Such experiments on intersensory localisation have a number of interesting characteristics which have profound implications for the control of movement. In particular they exhibit autokinesis and "ventriloquism" (see review and discussion in Howarth 1978).

Autokinesis was first studied by asking people to report any movement of a single spot of light in an otherwise completely dark room (see Howard and Templeton 1966, for a review of early work). Invariably it appears to wander in space in a relatively random fashion. This is a phenomenon of intersensory localisation because the light appears to move relative to the rest of the room or to the chair in which the subject sits. In the dark, the position of the chair is known by touch and by kinaesthesis, while the position of the light is judged visually (although ultimately even visual direction is judged in part kinaesthetically, because it depends on knowing the position of the eyes in their sockets and of the head relative to the rest of the body, as well as where on the retina the stimulus falls). Autokinesis is a demonstration of the instability of visual/kinaesthetic intersensory localisation. The same instability can be shown if the position of a source of sound is judged or if the subject is asked to judge the relative positions of a spot of light and a source of sound (Fisher 1961; Auerbach and Sperling 1974). One can even get the autokinetic phenomenon if people are asked to judge the relative positions of two limbs held out in space not touching each other.

The ventriloquism effect is a consequence of autokinesis and reflects one strategy for overcoming the loss of information which autokinesis produces. If the relative directions of two stimuli are not well known, the subject will use any additional information available to help to localise them. Autokinesis makes the relative direction of the sound of the ventriloquist's voice and its visually perceived source, the ventriloquist's head, very uncertain. The movement of the dummy's lips, aided by the quality of the ventriloquist's voice, suggests a possible alternative localisation of the voice, and this has no difficulty overcoming the imperfectly appreciated real relationship between the direction of the sound and its source. Exactly the same thing would happen if the ventriloquist's lips were seen to move, but in that case the assumed coincidence of visual and auditory signals would be veridical rather than an illusion.

The accuracy of intersensory localisation can be measured in a number of ways. One can measure the range of discrepancies created by autokinesis, but that requires a long period to elapse between opportunities to establish a veridical relationship. In many skilled activities there are relatively frequent opportunities to get the visual and kinaesthetic senses of direction to coincide. For example, in aiming at a target one may be able to see the target but not the hand in its starting position. Then, when the hand moves into view, and finally touches the target, visual information about the relative direction of limb and target can be used to correct any initial error due to autokinesis. Simultaneous sight of the hand and target during the course of a movement generates a visual error signal which may allow correction of the current movement (e.g. Paillard 1980), as well as correction of any error in the current relationship between visual and kinaesthetic information.

Our contention is that once the hand is withdrawn from the target and simultaneous vision of hand and target is lost, autokinesis will ensure that precise information about the relationship of the hand and target will deteriorate. We further suggest that this loss of information has important consequences for performance, and so it is important to know how the accuracy of absolute and relative spatial judgements varies over a relatively short time. Kinchla and Smyzer (1967) and Holding (1968) have shown that the inaccuracy of such judgements increases as time progresses from the last opportunity to bring the kinaesthetic and visual systems into synchronisation. There is, however, some debate about the precise time-course of this process. Kinchla and Smyzer suggested the standard deviation of such judgements was proportional to the square root of time, while Holding proposed a logarithmic relationship. These two functions are difficult to distinguish experimentally, but the first of them is easier to understand theoretically, since it implies a loss of information resulting from a random walk analogous to Brownian motion. In such systems the variance is proportional to time.

For our purposes, it is equally important to know something of the magnitude of these changes in perceptual knowledge about how we relate to the world. This can be estimated by measuring the standard deviation of repeated judgements of the relative direction of a visual and a kinaesthetically appreciated stimulus. Experiments of this kind by Fisher (1961) and by Auerbach and Sperling (1974) have found that the standard deviation of visual/kinaesthetic localisation (σ_{vk}) is approximately one degree, when considering repeated judgements with intervals of a few seconds between them.

Unfortunately, we know of no experiments which have plotted both the time course and the changes in the magnitude of these changes simultaneously. However, for our present purposes a value lying somewhere between a few seconds of arc (vernier acuity) and one degree for the standard deviation of visual/kinaesthetic localisation (σ_{vk}) over short periods (less than 10 s) is an important quantity which will be used repeatedly in the theory to be presented. To make the initial model simple, we will for the moment assume that σ_{vk} remains constant. This is clearly not true, so we will discuss in more detail later the consequences for performance of these changes in spatial knowledge.

A Theory of Speed-Error Trade-off in Relation to Variable Errors of Aiming

Our theory of speed-error trade-off in simple movements is based on *the assumption that accuracy of aiming, under open-loop conditions, is independent of movement time.* Earlier work by Woodworth (1899) and Vince (1948) on errors of stopping and by Keele and Posner (1968), where errors of aiming and stopping were confounded, suggested that this was likely to be the case. These earlier experiments had, like us, focussed on movement times in the range where visually mediated corrections would be expected in a closed-loop movement. More recently, interest in very rapid movements has led to experiments where movements are made so fast that it is unlikely that visually mediated corrections could be made (but see Carlton 1981, and Jagacinsky et al. 1980, for estimates of visual corrective reaction times much faster than hitherto measured). In very fast movements, typically completed in less than 200 ms, movement time *does* affect terminal accuracy, certainly for errors of stopping (Schmidt et al. 1979). The explanation for this effect is very different from the one which we will now develop, and although Wright and Meyer (1983) sought to extend the impulse variability model to account for *all* the variance of aiming performance at longer movement times, we feel that they were unjustified in doing so.

Impulse variability models offer a coherent way of thinking about the motor processes which affect the subject's ability to stop his or her arm. They are not concerned with errors made at right angles to the principal direction of movement, where the forces to control the arm are much less, and probably do not vary much with arm velocity. Consequently, we would predict that errors of aiming are independent of movement time, so long as the movement is completed faster than the corrective reaction time. At the moment, there are very little data to support this prediction, but we will discuss them later.

Our theory, on the other hand, is primarily concerned to account for aiming accuracy, measured as the standard deviation (σ_θ) of the angular error of aiming, in terms of the contribution to accuracy of corrections to a movement; these depend on visual information about the task being available to the subject. In the experiments to test our prediction that open-loop accuracy is independent of movement time, Beggs, Andrew, Baker, Dove, Fairclough and Howarth (1972) varied both distance and movement time, over a range from 350 to 1500 ms. Visually mediated corrections to the movement were prevented by switching off the illumination as soon as the movement started. Under these conditions, it was found that σ_a, the standard deviation of the hits around the target measured at right angles to the direction of movement (see Fig. 1), was proportional to the total distance moved (D) but largely independent of movement time, i.e.

$$\sigma_a = \sigma_\theta D. \tag{1}$$

This relationship is illustrated in Fig. 2.

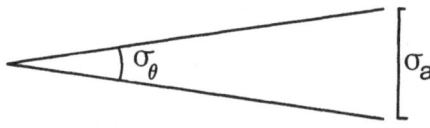

Fig. 2. The angular accuracy of aiming, σ_θ, and the resulting error of aiming, σ_a

Klapp (1975) found a similar effect, as did Schmidt et al. (1979). Meyer, Smith and Wright (1982), in their version of impulse-variability theory, show that precisely this result is predicted by their theory, but only for errors of stopping. Unlike our theory, however, their proportionality constant takes an arbitrary value. For our purposes, it is important to note that, in this experiment, σ_θ lies in the likely range identified from experiments on intersensory localisation, that is, somewhat less than one degree.

In an earlier experiment (Beggs and Howarth 1970) we showed that if the illumination is switched off during the movement of the hand towards a target, then the error on target is, as one would expect from Equation 1, proportional to the distance of the hand from the target when the illumination is switched off, d_c.

A small modification of Equation 1 to fit these data is needed:

$$\sigma_a = \sigma_\theta d_c, \tag{2}$$

where σ_θ again had a value somewhat less than one degree.

These two experiments support our basic assumption that, under open-loop conditions, aiming error is independent of movement time. They also appear to limit our theory of speed-error trade-off to situations where movements are under visual control. In other circumstances, where fast ballistic movements are made, other theories may be more appropriate (e.g. Kelso 1977; Klapp 1975; Meyer et al. 1982; Schmidt et al. 1979). It is not inconceivable that the motor processes which take precedence in fast movements will also operate in slower movements, with the result that our basic predictions may not account for all the variance in aiming performance. Nevertheless, we believe that in movements made in circumstances where visually mediated corrections may be used, our explanation, or one like it, will be necessary, and will account for most of the variance in the results obtained. In this, we differ from Wright and Meyer (1983).

Given the validity of Equations 1 and 2 under open-loop conditions, our theory assumes that any speed-accuracy relationship is determined by the effect which movement time has on the quantity d_c, the distance the hand travels after the last correction has been made to its trajectory, as shown in an idealised form in Fig. 3.

In practice, it is extremely difficult to observe discontinuities in the hand/arm system, probably because of damping. They have been measured in wrist rotations (Crossman and Goodeve 1963; Wright and Meyer 1983), where the degree of damping is much less. The same applies to very small movements, where discontinuities have also been observed (Jagacinski et al. 1980; Langolf, Chaffin and Foulke 1976).

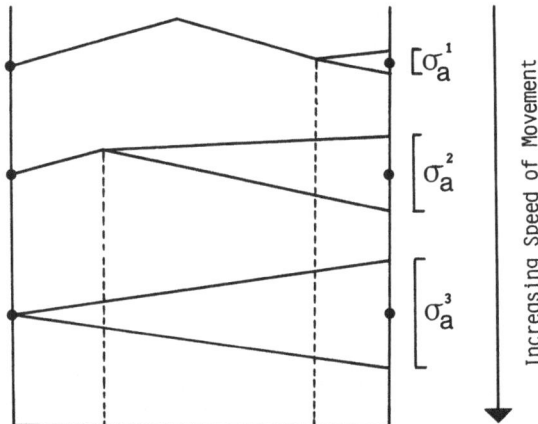

Fig. 3. The last correction made to movements of different speeds occurring at different distances from impact but with the same value of σ_θ

Our assumption is that slow movements leave time for the subject to fit one or more corrections into the movement, with the last of these corrections being made quite close to the target. Fast movements result in the last correction being made at some distance from the target, while for very fast movements there may not be time for any corrections at all, so that the movement becomes essentially ballistic (Keele and Posner 1968; Beggs and Howarth 1970). This hypothesis has to be distinguished from the simple iterative correction models of Crossman and Goodeve (1963) or Keele (1968).

In order to predict the relationship between movement time and accuracy, we need to understand the relationship between movement time and d_c, the distance from the target at which the last correction is made. To a first approximation, we assumed that this will occur when the hand is less than one corrective reaction time away from the target, since even if the need for a correction is realised, there will be no time to make one (Howarth et al. 1971). This assumption must be only approximately true, since the last correction may be made considerably further away of the need for additional corrections is realised too late; or, alternatively, the last correction may be made considerably nearer to the target in both space and time, when the need for a correction is recognised earlier, but cannot be organised until just before the hand hits the target. However, the assumption that the last correction is made, on average, at a distance corresponding to one corrective reaction time away from the target, was empirically justified (Beggs and Howarth 1970). In this experiment, when the lights were switched off as the hand approached a target, we found a mean value of 290 msec for the corrective reaction time in three of the faster movement time conditions. In another slower condition, a value of 165 msec was found. The higher value is close to that estimated by Keele and Posner (1968), while the lower value is close to that estimated recently by Jagacinski et al. (1980) and Carlton (1981).

There is considerable theoretical interest in the value of the corrective reaction time, and these different estimates are a problem for our theory. However, recent work by Jagacinski et al. (1980) showed that movements may have a series of corrective submovements, each with a decreasing duration. It would be interesting to speculate that our low value for the corrective reaction time, and the even shorter value reported by Carlton (1981), are late corrections in a series when the subject had time to introduce more than a single one. Keele (1981) regarded our theory as a "single correction" model; while it is the case that we regard the *final* correction to a movement as crucial, we have never precluded the possibility that under suitably long movement times more than one correction may be made.

For us, however, the real importance of the final correction is not its latency, but where in space it occurs in relation to the target. Howarth et al. (1971) measured the trajectory of the hand as it approaches the target. Trajectories were measured at different speeds by recording the time at which the hand broke an infrared beam set at different distances from the target, during an experiment in which the accuracy of movement was also measured. Figure 4 shows smooth curves drawn through data points averaged over several subjects. These trajector-

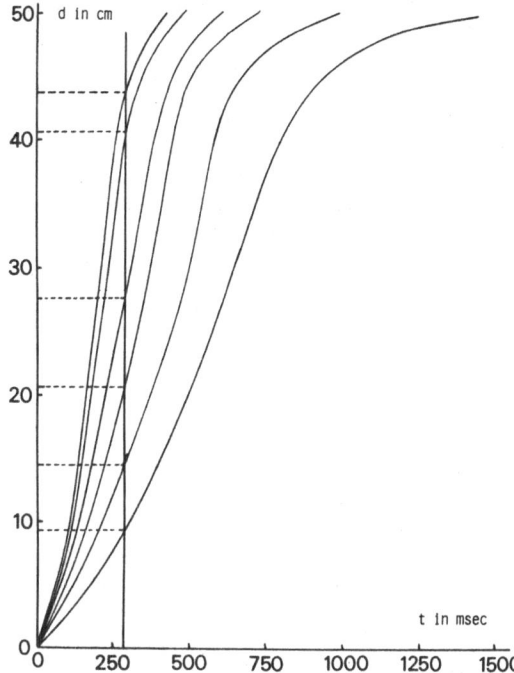

Fig. 4. Averaged approach curves at six different speeds. (Data from Howarth, Beggs, and Bowden 1971)

ies are plotted *backwards in time and in space* from the moment of impact on the target, which is thus represented by the origin.

This way of representing the results has the advantage of making it easy to read off the notional distance of the hand from the target when it is one corrective reaction time away from impact (d_c). This procedure is illustrated in Fig. 4 on the assumption that there is a single corrective reaction time of 290 ms, an estimate derived from the experiments of Beggs and Howarth (1970) conducted on the same apparatus. Howarth et al. (1971) then predicted the error on target using Equation 2. The empirical value of σ_a and the estimated values of d_c could be related by assuming a value of 36' for σ_θ. This, as we would expect, is somewhat less than the value of σ_{vk} obtained from the intersensory localisation experiments, where interstimulus judgements are separated by longer time intervals than in this experiment. However, like the value found in the non-visual aiming experiments reported above (Beggs et al. 1972), it is still close enough to justify our belief that intersensory localisation is a limiting factor in the accuracy of controlled movements.

As well as estimating d_c graphically as in Fig. 4, it can be calculated algebraically if the trajectories of Fig. 4 are described by a mathematical equation. This turns out to be comparatively easy. The final J-shaped segments of the trajectories can be represented by a power function

$$d = qt^n \ ,\tag{3}$$

where q is an arbitrary constant, d is the distance from the target and t is the time remaining before impact, as shown in Fig. 4; n is an empirically determined constant which, for the data shown in Fig. 4, is found to have a value of 1.4.

Surprisingly, and very conveniently, the curves of Figure 4 all turned out to have roughly the same shape; that is, the exponent n was independent of the total movement time. This has the advantage that the curves can all be collapsed onto a single curve, by scaling the values of t by the total movement time for given curve, T. In the same way, it should be possible, in principle, to scale the values of d by the total distance of movement (D) and thus derive a general expression for these approach trajectories.

Unfortunately, this scaling procedure cannot be done quite so simply since Equation 3 represents only the final decelerating portion of the trajectory and does not describe the initial accelerating portion. A complete mathematical treatment of such sigmoidal curves becomes very messy, especially when the trajectories are not symmetrical. This problem can be bypassed for the moment by postulating an imaginary distance D', which corresponds to the value of d in Equation 3 if t takes the value of T.

$$D' = q\,t^n\tag{3a}$$

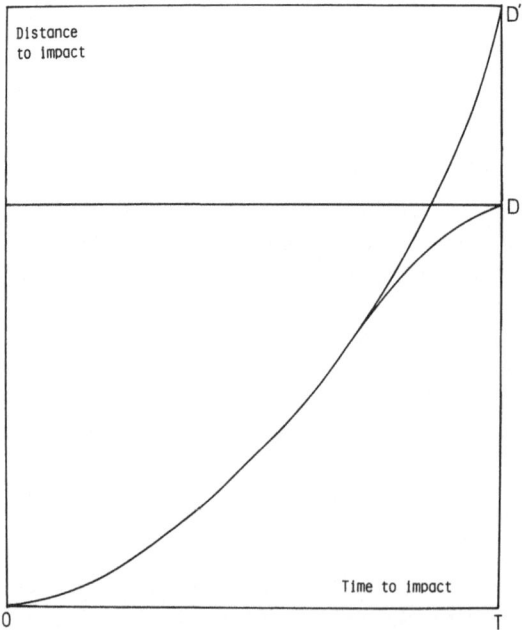

Fig. 5. The relationship of the real movement distance, D, to the computed distance, D'

The relationship between D' and D is shown in Figure 5. It clearly depends on the shape of the initial accelerating portion of the trajectory. For present purposes it can be expressed algebraically as

$$D' = KD.$$

Now, scaling d as a portion of D', represented as KD, and scaling t as a portion of T can be achieved by dividing Equation 3 by Equation 3a giving

$$\frac{d}{D} = K\left(\frac{t}{T}\right)^n. \tag{4}$$

If t is now given the value t_c (the corrective reaction time) as in Figure 3 we can calculate d_c

$$\frac{d_c}{D} = K\left(\frac{t_c}{T}\right)^n$$

or

$$d_c = KD\left(\frac{t_c}{T}\right)^n. \tag{5}$$

Putting this value of d_c in Equation 2 we get

$$\sigma_a = \sigma_\theta\, KD\left(\frac{t_c}{T}\right)^n. \tag{6}$$

This equation gives the desired relationship between movement time, T, and error σ_a.

However, it gives the misleading impression that as T becomes very large, i.e. when movements are very slow, σ_a will tend towards zero. In fact it does not. There is a limit on the accuracy of infinitely slow-aiming movements which is probably set by the uncontrollable tremor of the limb. This requires a slight modification to Equation 6. If we also measure tremor as a standard deviation (σ_t) then we can assume that it represents a source of variance, probably from the motor system, which is independent of σ_θ (and hence σ_a), which we are assuming comes from sensory systems. If these two sources of variance are really independent, their effects should be additive,

$$\sigma_\varepsilon^2 = \sigma_a^2 + \sigma_t^2, \tag{7}$$

where σ_ε^2 is the total measured variance in these experiments, σ_a^2 is the variance due to inaccuracies of aiming derived from Equation 6 and σ_t^2 is the tremor variance. Putting Equations 7 and 6 together we get

$$\sigma_\varepsilon^2 = K^2\, \sigma_\theta^2\, D^2 \left(\frac{t_c}{T}\right)^{2n} + \sigma_t^2. \tag{8}$$

Despite its apparent complexity, Equation 8 is conceptually very simple, as its derivation shows. It predicts the effect on the accuracy of aiming of both movement time and movement distance, the latter being one of the factors which Keele (1981) rightly identified as missing from our earlier version of the model.

Equation 8 is an idealised one, and its application is limited to paced aiming experiments, where variable errors of aiming are measured. Nevertheless, the underlying concepts are applicable to many other situations, where, for example, strategic changes to the movement itself can change this relationship between the main dependent and independent variables. These changes are not difficult to understand, but may be difficult to model, simply because of the rather complex mathematics involved.

The strength of Equation 8, or rather its basic method of derivation, is that every quantity, apart from the measured dependent and independent variables σ_ε^2, T and D, can be estimated in more than one type of experiment. The fundamental variables which we consider are σ_θ, t_c, σ_t, K and n.

σ_θ can be estimated from intersensory localisation experiments and from the accuracy of aiming in the dark (Fisher, 1961; Beggs et al., 1972), t_c can be estimated in many different ways (e.g. Beggs and Howarth, 1970; Keele and Posner, 1968; Vince, 1948), and σ_t can be measured by recording the uncontrollable tremor of the hand when we attempt to hold it still (Hick, 1952) and from the zero intercept when σ_ε^2 is plotted against $\left(\dfrac{1}{T}\right)^{2n}$.

Strategic changes in performance, which will depend on the precise nature of the task demands, appear to have their greatest effect on n (Beggs and Howarth 1972). Both n and K can be estimated from curve fitting on the relationship between σ_ε and speed of movement, but are best estimated from the shape of the trajectory of the hand as it approaches the target as shown in Fig. 4; n can be estimated by plotting $\log t$ against $\log d$, while K is best estimated from the kind of construction shown in Fig. 5 or by calculating D' as in Equation 3a.

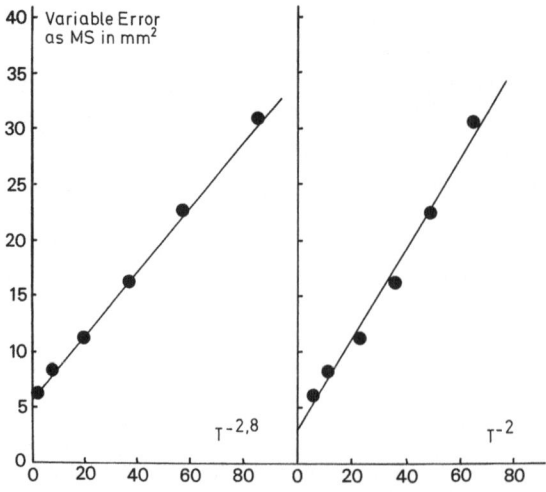

Fig. 6. Two possible relationships between error and movement speed

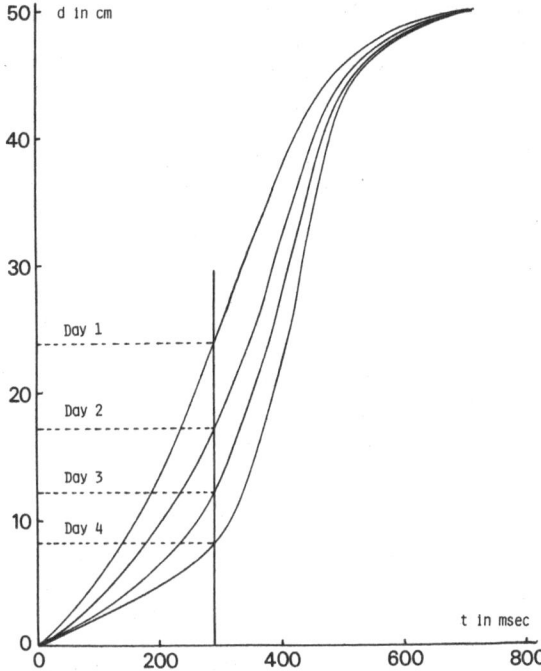

Fig. 7. Changes in approach curves with practice on successive days

Figure 6 shows the result of fitting the data of Howarth et al. (1971) to Equation 8.

Clearly the fit is very good, but in fact this kind of curve fitting is not a very accurate way to estimate n. Figure 6 also shows the same data plotted against $1/T^2$ rather than $1/T^{2.8}$. The fit is equally good, but the estimates of σ_t^2 are not accurate enough to help us discriminate between the two different estimates of n. In any case, curve-fitting is seldom a useful method for discriminating between rival theories.

Fortunately, there are other ways in which the underlying reality of Equation 8 can be tested. When subjects are given practice on this type of target-aiming task their accuracy improves. Beggs and Howarth (1972) have shown that a major factor in determining this improvement is a change in the trajectory of the hand as it approaches the target. Figure 7 shows some of their data.

It can be seen that practice reduced the distance of the hand from the target at the moment when only one corrective reaction time remained before impact. Beggs (1971) showed that these changes in the trajectories can be largely described by increases in the values of n, with much less important changes in the values of q in Equation 3. Early in practice, there may be almost no deceleration as the hand approaches the target and n will have a value close to 1.0. Later in practice the value of n increases until it approaches a value of 2.0, which corresponds to a constant deceleration (i.e. a parabola), causing the hand to stop smoothly, as it reaches the target, rather than crash into it. In the final phase of practice, n can take values up to 3.2. Practice also increases the speed of initial acceleration and this change is partly accounted for by changes in q.

We have recently found similar changes to trajectories in an unpaced aiming task. However, it still remains to be determined what proportion of the changes in aiming accuracy are due to the change in the trajectory of the hand, or indeed to show conclusively that the function relating speed and accuracy changes in exactly the same way as the change in the function describing the trajectory of the hand as it approaches the target.

Finally, it has been well demonstrated by many workers (Rashevsky 1959; Drury 1971; Beggs, Sakstein, and Howarth 1974) that for tasks such as driving a car or a forklift truck, or walking along a narrow beam of wood, where the speed of movement is constant (rather than changing, as it does when the arm decelerates towards a target) accuracy is inversely proportional to speed (i.e. σ_a is proportional to $1/T$). This is what would be expected if n takes a value of 1.0 in Equation 6 or Equation 8.

Fitting the Theory to the Data

One of the problems of working in this area is that different backgrounds have generated different interests which address different questions about motor performance. The resulting theories, and the data which accompany them, seem incompatible. For example, certain sorts of existing experimental data cannot easily be fitted by any one theory. This could be regarded as sufficient grounds for rejecting those theories which fail to account for those data. But if theories in this area were rejected because they were unable to explain all the data, no theories would survive. While accepting that it is the function of theories to make sense of data, it must also be admitted that data tend to be messy, to be reported in ways which are inappropriate, and in many cases to be downright misleading. In an ideal world, theories should be tested against clean data, obtained in circumstances which are appropriate to the theory. In addition, if different mechanisms and different control strategies are likely to operate under different circumstances, then it is unreasonable to expect the same theory to apply to all of them. Indeed, any theory which did apply equally well in all circumstances would be rather unconvincing. We believe that the major problem in testing any theory of motor control is to decide which subset of the data should be explained.

Accordingly, the available evidence will now be reviewed and classified. Initially only data concerning the relationship between movement time and variable errors of aiming will be considered, since these are the data which are best fitted by the theory we have detailed above. However, we will also consider data on the effect of movement time on variable errors of stopping. These show some differences from the errors of aiming, but the differences are fairly easily explained.

Data on the effect of movement time on constant errors will also be discussed. Some of these data are quite difficult for the theory being put forward here, because they confound variable and constant errors. This makes it almost impossible to understand what was really happening, let alone model it.

Finally, the differences between paced and unpaced experiments will be discussed. In relation to variable errors the differences are minor and relatively easily explained. In relation to constant errors, the differences are considerable and require a radically different type of explanation.

Variable Errors of Aiming

The lines on Fig. 8 show the idealised form of the data we would expect from the theory presented in the last section and from Equations 1–8, while the points on Fig. 8 represent real data drawn from several sources. There are four different regions in the idealised data.

Region 1 contains open-loop data. Open-loop conditions may be achieved either for very fast movements for which there is no time to make a correction even if an error of aiming is detected or for slow movements during which it is impossible to detect any errors. This latter condition is usually achieved by switching off the illumination as soon as the movement starts. The idealised form of the data in Region 1 is adequately described by Equation 1:

$$\sigma_a = \sigma_\theta D$$

For slow movements, errors will be undetected only when the target ceases to be visible during the movement (Beggs et al. 1972; Keele and Posner 1968; Vince 1948; Woodworth 1899). When both hand and target are visible, then accurate

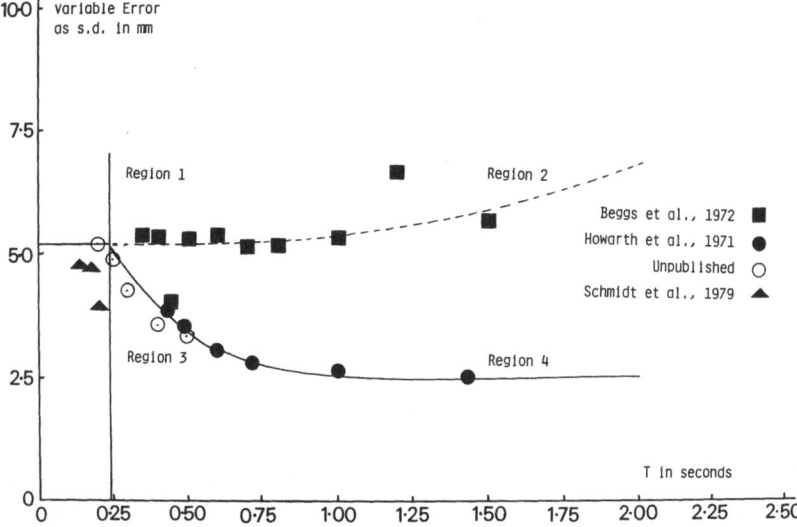

Fig. 8. The hypothetical relationship between movement speed and errors of aiming under open- and closed-loop conditions, with some typical data

corrections to the movement are possible, as is described below for Region 3. When only the target is visible, and the position of the hand is perceived kinaesthetically, then corrections to the movement can still take place, but with less accuracy than when the error signal is entirely visual (unpublished data, Beggs and Howarth).

Region 2 also contains open-loop data but for movement times very much longer than those in Region 1. Work by Woodworth (1899) and Holding (1968) suggests that the increase in error in this region is due to a kind of forgetting process during the delay between completing one aiming movement and starting another. Both Woodworth and Holding manipulated this interval independently of movement time although in repetitive aiming it is of course equal to the movement time of the aiming phase of the movement. Recent work by Beggs (1984) has confirmed their findings.

It is an important part of our theory that we assume this increase in σ_θ to be the same as the increase in autokinesis (σ_{vk}) with time, although until now, we have assumed, for simplicity in model building, that σ_θ remains constant. A central assumption is that during the time from the completion of one movement to the completion of the next, visual and kinaesthetic spaces have the opportunity to drift apart. We would thus expect to see an effect on performance, i.e.

$$\sigma_\theta = j \sqrt{t_m + t_i},\qquad\qquad(9)$$

where j is a proportionality constant, t_m is movement time, and t_i the intertrial interval. The square-root function describes the timecourse of a random-walk process.

Kinchla and Smyzer (1967) presented evidence of the diffusion of memory for the visual position of a stimulus, although in their experiments no movements were made. In such conditions we know that when t_i is zero, or close to it, the error of localization can be as little as a few seconds of angle (vernier or movement acuity). In aiming experiments, where movements are made fairly rapidly, we may need to add a further constant to Equation 9, which represents either the variance due to the activity of planning and executing a movement or some inescapable additional error due to the necessary intersensory comparisons, or both.

In Fisher's experiments (Fisher 1961), no error due to intersensory comparison was found (see discussion in Howarth 1978), so it is likely that the constancy of σ_θ for short movement times is due to additional variance introduced by the planning and execution of a movement, σ^2_m. Thus the relationship of σ_θ to movement time becomes

$$\sigma^2_\theta = j^2 (t_m + t_i) + \sigma^2_m,\qquad\qquad(10)$$

The data points from Beggs et al. (1972) show an upturn for longer movement times which is consistent with Equation 10. The constancy of σ_θ for small values of t_m (and t_i) must occur when $j^2 (t_m + t_i)$ becomes small compared with σ^2_m. This seems to occur when $(t_m + t_i)$ is less than about 2 or 3 s.

Region 3 shows the idealised form of the data for closed loop, visually controlled aiming, where movement times are longer than the corrective reaction time. It is to this region that the theory represented by Equation 6 applies. The data points in this region are from the experiments of Howarth et al. (1971), but rescaled with respect to movement distance. Also shown are some previously unreported data from our laboratory which covered movement times faster than those reported by Howarth et al. (1971).

Region 4 also shows the idealised form of the data for visually controlled aiming, but for much longer movement times than in Region 3. Here the accuracy of aiming again becomes independent of speed, probably because it is limited by tremor in the limb. The data points in this region are also taken from the experiments of Howarth et al. (1971).

The transition from Region 3 to Region 4 is described by Equations (7) and (8).

A point of particular interest is the transition from Region 1 to Region 4 which, in visually controlled aiming, should occur at the corrective reaction time. None of the movement times reported by us have been fast enough to investigate this region, but some data from Schmidt et al. (1979) shown in Figure 8 seem to support our rather surprising prediction that errors of aiming are not related to movement time when the movement time is less than the corrective reaction time. Analysis of some new data from our laboratory showed that there was no significant increase in visually controlled errors of aiming when movement times are decreased from 250 to 200 ms, exactly as we predicted. These data are shown on Fig. 8. Errors of stopping, however, did increase, as impulse variability theory predicts. It will be important to investigate these boundary conditions more rigorously.

It is clear from other work on corrective reaction times (cf. Keele and Posner 1968) that t_c may be somewhat less than our own estimate of 290 ms. In fact, such a reduction in t_c on Fig. 8 to a figure of about 200 ms fits the observed data rather better. More recent estimates of t_c have suggested that it may be even lower. For example, Carlton (1981) suggested that it could be as low as 135 ms. The task he used was single-shot unpaced aiming, and he reports that at about 290 ms into the movement a change in the trajectory was observed. This was in spite of the subject being unable to see most of his movement. The implicit assumption made by Carlton, like Paillard (1980), is that movements are corrected on the basis of a visual/visual error signal. Some work in our own laboratory, which we hope soon to publish, confirms our own view that the error signal can be intersensory. If this is the case, sight of the hand approaching the target is not essential for *control,* but is important in order to keep the visual and kinaesthetic spaces in synchrony. What Carlton's data may show is a correction occurring with a latency of about the order of our own estimate of the corrective reaction time, based on a intersensory error signal.

Lower estimates for the visual correlative reaction time have also been suggested by Jagacinski et al. (1980). There is reason to suppose, however, that their lower estimates are applicable only to very slow movements and may represent second corrections with a shorter latency. Hence, they are not applicable to the point of inflection in Fig. 8, below which a further reduction in movement time ceases to increase error.

Variable Errors of Stopping

In contrast to errors of aiming, which are measured perpendicular to the direction of movement, errors of stopping are measured in the direction of the movement itself. Figure 9 shows some data on variable errors of stopping. The idealised form of the data in Fig. 8 is repeated in this figure for comparison. There are three main points to be noted about the real data points for variable errors of stopping.

Region 1 shows that open-loop errors of stopping are as independent of speed as are errors of aiming for movement times longer than about 0.5 s. However, they are approximately 25% greater than the variable errors of aiming. This is shown most clearly in the data of Beggs et al. (1972), where errors of aiming, and errors of stopping, were measured simultaneously for subjects aiming at a dot target.

Region 2 shows that errors of stopping also increase with long movement times, as they do for errors of aiming. Data from Beggs et al. (1972), Vince (1948) and Woodworth (1899) all show an upturn for longer movement times.

Region 3 shows that errors of stopping for visually controlled movements fall rather more sharply than errors of aiming as the duration of movement is increased. There are at least two possible reasons for this. One is that for slow movements the distinction between errors of stopping and errors of aiming becomes less meaningful, particularly for movements which are not constrained to a single plane. As one approaches a target on a table, the initial movement may be in the direction in which errors of stopping are measured, but, as the movement slows down over the target and the hand descends towards it at the last mo-

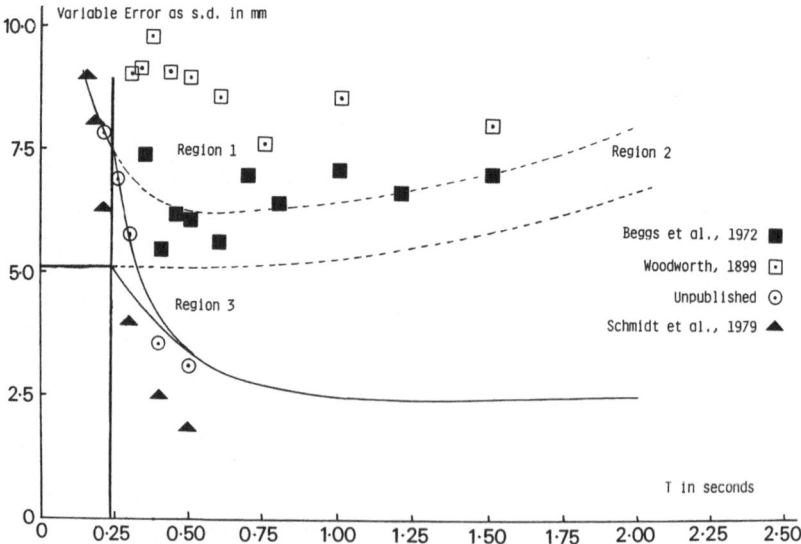

Fig. 9. The hypothetical relationship between movement speed and errors of stopping under open- and closed-loop conditions, with some typical data

ment, the final approach may be at right angles to the table and to the direction in which the error is measured. Thus, for fast speeds, visually controlled errors of stopping, like open-loop errors of stopping, may be 25% greater than errors of aiming. But, for longer movement times, this difference may disappear.

A second reason why errors of stopping are more critically affected by movement time than errors of aiming is that they do not level off for the very fastest movements. Schmidt et al. (1979) and Meyer et al. (1982) have both produced data of this kind for which error appears to be proportional to the velocity of movement.

$$\sigma_S = \frac{K}{T} \tag{11}$$

Schmidt et al. and Meyer et al. are not in agreement about the precise details of the model for impulse variability theory, although both have suggested that increases in error are due to the greater variability of the large muscle forces required for rapid acceleration and deceleration of the arm. The final version of the theory will probably be very different from the present discussion on visually controlled movement. But there need be no conflict between these different theories because they refer to very different phenomena obtained under very different experimental conditions.

Impulse variability theory is primarily concerned to explain errors of stopping. As we have seen, errors of stopping, even in conditions where visually mediated corrections would be expected, are generally higher than errors of aiming. It may be that in the former we see the operation of both a perceptual and a motor component.

Effect of Pacing

Figure 10 shows some comparisons of variable errors of aiming under paced conditions (taken from Howarth et al. 1971) and some as yet unpublished data from an unpaced aiming task. (We hope to publish these in detail at a later date.) In the paced condition the subject aimed repeatedly at a line target in time with a metronome. In the unpaced condition , the subject aimed at targets of varying widths as fast as possible while still keeping within the target. However, accuracy was measured as the standard deviation of hits about the mean of the distribution of hits within the target. In Fig. 10, it can be seen that unpaced movements are more accurate at slow speeds than are paced movements.

Newell (1980) has suggested that pacing requires some effort to be accurate in time and that this detracts from the ability to be accurate in space, which might explain why unpaced aiming is more accurate than paced aiming for reasonably slow movements.

Newell is almost certainly right, but his explanation can be elaborated a little in the context of the present theory. Unpaced movements give the subject a better opportunity to adjust the trajectory of the hand so as to reduce error to a

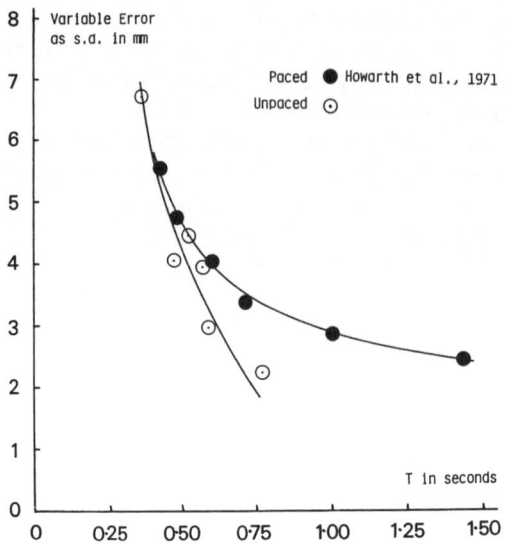

Fig. 10. The change in the relationship of error to movement speed as a function of the paced and unpaced movement paradigms. (From Howarth, Beggs, and Bowden 1971; and unpublished)

minimum. The best way to do this should be to get as near to the target as possible before the last correction is made, which should show up as a higher value of n in Equation 4). In the paced condition, n took a value of 1.4, which remained constant at different movement times. In the unpaced experiment, n varied between 2.46 and 1.75 as the target width increased from 5 to 50 mm and as movement time decreased accordingly. We consider that these data describe a strategic adaptation to the task demands by the subject, just as our earlier data (Beggs et al. 1972) showed a similar change in trajectories as a subject became more skilled and more accurate.

However, the data in Fig. 10 suggest that even this explanation is incomplete, since the accuracy of very slow unpaced movements seems to become better than one would expect if it were limited by tremor. However, if the hand is held over a target trembling, but not under time pressure, it may be possible to choose the best moment to drop the hand onto the target, provided the tremor is not too rapid. Subjectively this seems to be what happens for unpaced movements, but no experimental test of this "selection from tremor" hypothesis has yet been devised.

Recently, Wright and Meyer (1983) have advanced a very different explanation for the difference between paced and unpaced movements. Using a version of the impulse variability model developed by them (Meyer et al. 1982), they predicted, and found, that in a paced wrist rotation aiming task, error and movement time were linearly related. They included movement times longer than any visual corrective reaction time estimate.

Their experiment was very different from the paradigm that we have used and seek to model. The subject had to halt the movement himself, and so they were measuring errors of stopping. In any case, the fact that a target physically stops the movement may in itself be important. Second, the movements made by their subjects were not repetitive, but were single-shot attempts to meet a criterion time. Under these conditions, subjects may operate rather differently. Finally, they did not directly test the possibility that their subjects were aiming ballistically, "choosing" not to use the available visual information to update their movements (Zelaznik et al. 1981). For these reasons, and because they dealt inadequately with the comparison between our work, that of Kerr and Langolf (1977) and their own, we do not regard this experiment as a serious difficulty for our approach based on strategy changes to hand trajectories.

Constant Errors

All the data and theories presented so far have been related to variable errors of movement. Constant errors have been ignored. One justification for this is that constant errors of aiming can be negligibly small (Beggs 1971). Another is that constant errors are very complexly related to the direction and length of movement, and these relationships seem to have no relationship to any of the present theories, although they are extensively discussed in relation to motor memory (Laabs and Simmons 1981). The principal empirical results taken from Beggs' (1971) review are:

1. Constant errors tend to be undershoots for large movements and overshoots for short movements.
2. They tend to be further from the body than targets which are near to the body and closer to the body than targets which are far from the body. (This can be independent of the length and direction of movement.)
3. For radial movements away from the body, errors tend to be towards the sagittal plane.
4. Each of these different types of error is greater for faster movements and for poor levels of sensory control.

No adequate explanation has ever been offered for these results, nor is it possible to use data on constant errors to test any of the theories of control of movement which have been considered in this paper.

   In the past, data have tended to be rather loosely reported, so that they cannot be used to test theories adequately. It is particularly inappropriate to use performance measures which confuse constant and variable errors. Unfortunately, the worst of all possible experimental paradigms in this respect is the one which has been used most frequently, i.e. that originally developed by Paul Fitts (1954). Fitts used several versions of an unpaced task, in which subjects were asked either to move backwards and forwards as quickly as possible between two strip targets of fixed width, or to place pegs as quickly as possible into holes of a fixed size. He found a logarithmic relationship between the speed of movement and the width of the target or the diameter of the hole:

$$T = a + b \log_2 \frac{2A}{W},$$

(12)

where T is the total movement time, A the amplitude of the movement and W the width of the target, while a and b are arbitrary constants. Fitts related this empirical expression to information theory, regarding $\log_2 2A/W$ as a measure of the information content of the movement.

Because of its similarity to other functions relating reaction times or movement times to measures of information, Equation 12 and Fitts' paradigm have played a dominant role in studies of speed-accuracy trade-off (see, for example, Welford 1968).

The information theory account has been severely criticised by several writers, including Howarth (1978) and Howarth and Beggs (1981), who pointed out that Fitts' original formulation should apply also to open-loop movements. Hence, the absence of any effect of movement time on the accuracy of such movements (see Figs. 8, 9) is very strong evidence against the generalisation of Fitts' *theory* to movements which cannot be corrected visually.

Alternative explanations for Fitt's law have attempted to take a control-theory perspective of closed-loop aiming. Crossman and Goodeve (1963) developed an explanation of the logarithmic function, assuming that either visually or kinaesthetically mediated error signals could result in corrections and that these would be made at fairly regular intervals until no more time remained. In that respect their theory was like the one proposed by Keele (1968), who considered that corrections would rely on a visual error signal. Assuming that movement error will be reduced by a constant fraction each time a correction is made leads to the same logarithmic function which Fitts and others have observed.

Keele (1981) makes a number of criticisms of this iterative correction model of movement control. The most important problem with the approach is that the underlying assumption, that terminal accuracy is a function of the *number* of corrections, cannot be reconciled with the fact that corrective reaction times are so long in relation to movement times. There may be time to fit one, two or perhaps three corrections into a movement; terminal accuracies, however, do not vary in a stepwise fashion with changes in movement time.

We consider that it is very unlikely that the experimental situation used by Fitts yields data which can be given any simple theoretical explanation. The unpaced tasks used by Fitts require the subject to make a movement with sufficiently small constant error and/or a sufficiently small variable error. It is now almost certain that movement time affects constant errors in different ways in different situations and that in none of them is there any simple relationship between constant and variable errors (Beggs 1971). The logarithmic function observed by Fitts and others may be practically useful, but it is profoundly unhelpful for any attempt at a theoretical explanation of movement errors.

A Further Elaboration of the Theory

The theory presented earlier can be regarded as an account of how subjects make strategic adaptations to the decay of spatial information. Because accuracy of localisation has been lost due to the decay process described by Equation 9, corrections are made whenever the error is large enough to be detected. This raises two further questions:

1. Why is spatial information lost so quickly?
2. Are there any other strategic adaptations to the difficulties created by its loss?

Howarth (1978) has suggested that spatial information decays because we do not have enough storage space in the brain to remember it. He argued that the complex articulation of the body would require a very large amount of storage space if all possible positions of all the limbs were to be recorded and remembered, together with the necessary information about how to get from one position to another. We do not navigate our bodies by the use of accurate maps and the kind of super-efficient dead reckoning which inertial navigation instruments make possible for nuclear submarines. Instead we use methods more like those of the ancient navigators. We make accurate observations when we can locate our bodies in space by vision, which is our most accurate sense, and when the other spatial senses can be calibrated against vision or against each other. But this information is rapidly lost, and we navigate by using "rules of thumb" (literally sometimes) which have worked in the past and which reduce the risks entailed by our poor memory for spatial localisation.

Recent work by Thomson (1983) has shown how people can locomote without visual guidance towards remote targets for only about 8 sec before beginning to make large errors. Thereafter, they are unable to relate themselves to their surroundings and begin to make navigational errors of the type we would predict. Many other aspects of motor behaviour can be seen as strategic adaptations to the underlying difficulty of this loss of spatial information necessary for controlling our actions. For example, the warming-up period which is necessary for all high-level skills has the effect of increasing the blood supply to the muscles and loosening the joints, but it may also enable us to relearn what it feels like to do it right and to recalibrate the senses which are responsible for fine tuning. Although there is a literature on warm-up effects, no-one has tested a prediction which flows from our hypothesis. It should be possible to show that warming-up activity increases the accuracy of intersensory localisation.

There are many studies of adaptation to distortions of spatial relations. The earlier studies were of the effects of total inversion of the visual field (Stratton 1896; Snyder and Pronko 1952; Kohler 1962), but more recent studies have been of the effect of wearing prisms which merely deviate the apparent location of visual objects by a few degrees (e.g. Held 1961). We can adapt very rapidly to these minor deviations, and Howarth (1978) has suggested that the mechanisms which make this adaptation possible are the same as those which enable us to overcome the equally large deviations of visual direction which can develop naturally as a result of autokinesis.

Studies of adaptation to deviations of visual direction have shown that it can be exceedingly specific. For example, both Harris (1963) and Hamilton (1964) have shown that learning to point correctly with one hand does not, by transfer, lead to any improvement in pointing with the other hand. This specificity of learning is what one would expect if we are not attempting to know all the relationships between all parts of the body.

The loss of accuracy in delayed aiming, which is described by Equation 9, may also be responsible for some other aspects of the timing of skilled movements which are usually explained in the language of information theory. Since Merkel first investigated them in 1880, it has been known that choice reaction times are longer, the greater the number of choices.

Hick (1952) showed that the relationship was a logarithmic one:

$$T = K \log_2 (N + 1),$$

(13)

where N is the number of choices. He suggested that $\log (N+1)$ is a measure of the information contained in each choice. He used $N+1$ rather than N since the subjects always had the possibility of making no response.

This information theory account of choice reaction times has been challenged many times. Recently we (Howarth and Beggs 1981) have suggested that the crucial factor is the loss of spatial information over time and that Equation 13 reflects the same phenomenon as Equation 9. It is, of course, extremely difficult to differentiate between a logarithmic and square root function. Beggs (1984) has recently produced evidence that the critical factor which determines both aiming accuracy and response latency is not choice, but the time since the subject made the last movement or response. When a movement or response is made, the subject has an opportunity to calibrate the kinaesthetic, motor and visual systems against each other. During the delay between successive movements, this information is lost again due to autokinesis. Thus, the continual updating of intersensory information is essential, not only to improve accuracy, but also to make it possible for us to act quickly.

Conclusion

The theory we have presented holds that for movement times between about 200 and 2000 ms, variable errors of aiming are largely determined by the subject's efforts to get as close to the target as possible before the last correction has been made to the direction of the hand. It follows from this that the relationship between movement time and error is the same as the relationship between time and distance as the hand approaches the target. We believe that the available evidence strongly supports this view, but many further predictions could be made and tested.

Our analysis of the way in which data on movement have been collected and reported in the past suggests that the many other functions describing the relationship of movement time to terminal accuracy do not contradict our own for one or more of the following reasons:

1. They are concerned with constant errors rather than variable errors.
2. They relate to errors of stopping rather than errors of aiming.

3. The movement times are outside the range used by us.
4. Correction of movement is prevented by lack of time or appropriate information.

These different conditions inevitably lead to the operation of different mechanisms with different relationships between speed and error.

The underlying reason why subjects attempt to get as close to the target as possible before making the last correction to the hand is because of the comparative inaccuracy with which we are able to sense the relationship between different parts of our bodies and between our bodies and objects in space around us. These inaccuracies are a consequence of, and are compounded by, the loss of intersensory information over time. This is directly demonstrated in the autokinetic phenomenon and easily observed in the reduced accuracy of very slow, uncorrected movements. In visually corrected movements lasting between 200 and 2000 ms, getting as close to the target as possible before making the last correction to the trajectory of the hand is the best available strategy. The operation of this strategy determines the precise relationship between movement time and terminal error, and, indeed, many other aspects of such movements. Under other circumstances, other mechanisms and strategies become dominant. Evidence favouring other theories in other circumstances cannot be regarded as evidence against the theory presented here.

References

Auerbach, C., and Sperling, P. (1974). A common auditory-visual space: Evidence for its reality. Perception and Psychophysics, 16, 129–135.

Bainbridge, L., and Sanders, M. (1972). The generality of Fitt's Law. Journal of Experimental Psychology, 96, 130–133.

Beggs, W. D. A. (1971). Movement control. Unpublished PhD Thesis, University of Nottingham.

Beggs, W. D. A. (1984). The accuracy and speed of repeated responses. Psychological Research, 46, 87–105.

Beggs, W. D. A., and Howarth, C. I. (1970). Movement control in a repetitive motor task. Nature, 225, 752–753.

Beggs, W. D. A., and Howarth, C. I. (1972). The movement of the hand towards a target. Quarterly Journal of Experimental Psychology, 24, 448–453.

Beggs, W. D. A., Andrew, J. A., Baker, M. L., Dove, S. R., Fairclough, I., and Howarth, C. I. (1972). The accuracy of nonvisual aiming. Quarterly Journal of Experimental Psychology, 24, 515–523.

Beggs, W. D. A., Sakstein, R., and Howarth, C. I. (1974). The generality of a theory of intermittent control of accurate movements. Ergonomics, 17, 757–768.

Bizzi, E., Polit, A., and Morasso, P. (1976). Mechanisms underlying achievement of final head position. Journal of Neurophysiology, 39, 435–444.

Carlton, L. G. (1981). Processing visual feedback information for movement control. Journal of Experimental Psychology: Human Perception and Performance, 7, 1019–1030.

Crossman, E. R. F. W., and Goodeve, P. J. (1963). Feedback control of hand-movement and Fitt's Law. Paper presented at the meeting of the Experimental Psychology Society, Oxford, 1963. Quarterly Journal of Experimental Psychology, 1983, 35 A, 251–278.

Drury, C. G. (1971). Movements with lateral restraint. Ergonomics, 14, 293–303.

Fisher, G. H. (1961). Autokinesis in the spatial senses. Bulletin of the British Psychological Society, 44, 16–17 A.

Fitts, P. M. (1954). The information capacity of the human motor system controlling the amplitude of movement. Journal of Experimental Psychology, 47, 381–391.

Hamilton, C. R. (1964). Intermanual transfer of adaptation to prisms. American Journal of Psychology, 77, 457–462.

Harris, C. S. (1963). Adaptation to displaced vision: Visual, motor or proprioceptive change? Science, 140, 812–813.

Held, R. (1961). Exposure history as a factor in maintaining stability of perception and co-ordination. Journal of Nervous and Mental Disorders, 132, 26–32.

Hick, W. E. (1952). On the rate of gain of information. Quarterly Journal of Experimental Psychology, 4, 11–26.

Holding, D. H. (1968). Accuracy of delayed aiming responses. Psychonomic Science, 12 (4), 125–126.

Howard, I. P., and Templeton, W. B. (1966). Human spatial orientation. New York: Wiley.

Howarth, C. I. (1978). Strategies in the control of movement. In G. Underwood (Ed.), Strategies of information processing. London: Academic.

Howarth, C. I., and Beggs, W. D. A. (1981). Discrete movements. In D. M. Holding (Ed.) Human skills. New York: Wiley.

Howarth, C. I., Beggs, W. D. A., and Bowden, J. (1971). The relationship between speed and accuracy of movement aimed at a target. Acta Psychologica, 35, 207–218.

Jagacinski, R. J., Repperger, D. W., Moran, M. S., Ward, S. L., and Glass, B. (1980). Fitts Law and the microstructure of rapid discrete movements. Journal of Experimental Psychology: Human Perception and Performance, 6, 309–320.

Keele, S. W. (1968). Movement control in skilled motor performance. Psychological Bulletin, 70, 387–403.

Keele, S. W. (1981). Behavioral analysis of movement. In: Brooks V. (ed.) Handbook of physiology: The nervous system: Vol. 2. Motor control. Baltimore: American Physiological Society.

Keele, S. W., and Posner, M. I. (1968). Processing of visual feedback in rapid movements. Journal of Experimental Psychology, 77 (1) 155–158.

Kelso, J. A. S. (1977). Motor control mechanisms underlying human movement reproduction. Journal of Experimental Psychology: Human Perception and Performance, 3, 529–543.

Kerr, B. A., and Langolf, G. D. (1977). Speed of aiming movements. Quarterly Journal of Experimental Psychology, 29, 475–481.

Kinchla, R. A., and Smyzer, F. (1967). A diffusion model of perceptual memory. Perception and Psychophysics, 2, 219–229.

Klapp, S. T. (1975). Feedback versus motor programming in the control of aimed movements. Journal of Experimental Psychology: Human Perception and Performance, 1, 147–153.

Kohler, I. (1962). Experiments with goggles. Scientific American, 206, 62–86.

Laabs, G. J., and Simmons, R. W. (1981). Motor memory. In D. H. Holding (Ed.) Human skills. New York: Wiley.

Langolf, G. D., Chaffin, D. B., and Foulke, J. A. (1976). An investigation of Fitts Law using a wide range of movement amplitudes. Journal of Motor Behavior, 8, 113–128.

Meyer, D. E., Smith, J. E. K., and Wright, C. E. (1982). Models for the speed and accuracy of aimed movements. Psychological Review, 89, 449–482.

Newell, K. M. (1980). The speed-accuracy paradox in movement control: error of time and space. In G. E. Stelmach and J. Requin (Eds.) Tutorials in motor behavior. Amsterdam: Elsevier-North Holland.

Paillard, J. (1980). The multichanneling of visual cues and the organization of a visually guided response. In: G. E. Stelmach and J. Requin (Eds.) Tutorials in motor behavior. Amsterdam: Elsevier-North Holland.

Rashevsky, N. (1959). Mathematical biophysics of automobile driving. Bulletin of Mathematical Biophysics, 21, 375–385.

Schmidt, R. A., Zelaznik, H., Hawkins, B., Frank, J. S., and Quinn, J. T. (1979). Motor output variability: A theory for the accuracy of rapid motor acts. Psychological Review, 86, 415–451.

Snyder, R. W., and Pronko, N. H. (1952). Vision with spatial inversion. Wichita, Kansas: McCormick-Armstrong.

Stratton, G. M. (1896). Some preliminary experiments in vision without inversion of the retinal image. Psychological Review, 3, 611–617; (1897) 4, 182–187, 341–360, 363–481.

Thomson, J. A. (1983). Is visual monitoring necessary in visually guided motion? Journal of Experimental Psychology: Human Perception and Performance, 9, 427–443.

Vince, M. A. (1948). Corrective movements in a pursuit task. Quarterly Journal of Experimental Psychology, 1, 85–106.

Welford, A. T. (1968). Fundamentals of skill. London: Methuen.

Wright, C. E., and Meyer, D. E. (1983). Conditions for a linear speed-accuracy trade-off in aimed movements. Quarterly Journal of Experimental Psychology, 35 A, 279–296.

Woodworth, R. S. (1899). Accuracy of voluntary movement. Psychological Review, Monograph Supplement 3 (No 3), 1–114.

Zelaznik, H. N., Shapiro, D. C., and McClosky, D. (1981). Effects of a secondary task on the accuracy of single aiming movements. Journal of Experimental Psychology: Human Perception and Performance, 7, 1007–1018.

The Movement Speed-Accuracy Relationship in Space-Time

P. A. HANCOCK and K. M. NEWELL

Contents

Introduction

In this chapter we synthesize extant descriptions of the movement speed-accuracy relationship and develop, from these orientations, a space-time approach to movement accuracy. This new space-time perspective provides a cohesive account of spatial and temporal movement error functions in the face of changing kinematics. The space-time function is posited as a statistical manifestation of the organismic, environmental, and task constraints inherent to the given action.

The relationship between movement speed and accuracy is an issue that has enjoyed considerable theoretical and empirical activity in the psychological domain. Since the seminal experimental work of Fullerton and Cattell (1892), descriptions of the movement speed-accuracy relationship have focused almost exclusively on errors in a single or dual spatial dimension (e.g., Beggs and Howarth 1970; Crossman and Goodeve 1963; Fitts 1954; Woodworth 1899). Moreover, these formulations have been confined to spatial errors which have been produced principally at or toward the upper end of the velocity continuum for prescribed movement amplitude and target tolerance conditions. A recent account of the movement-speed timing-accuracy relationship has examined a wide range of movement velocities but has also been limited to tasks with criteria in only one or two spatial dimensions (Newell 1980; Newell, Hoshizaki, Carlton, and Halbert 1979; Newell, Carlton, Carlton, and Halbert 1980).

The above formulations of the movement speed-accuracy function have accounted for restricted segments of the overall speed-accuracy relationship. We propose that a complete description of this relationship should examine both spatial and temporal components of movement across the complete range of movement generation available to the human performer in the accomplishment of discrete motoric acts. The chapter shows that when both temporal and spatial errors are measured in the same plane of motion, the movement-speed error functions for each moment of the error distribution are consonant.

This space-time approach to movement speed-accuracy provides an enhanced perspective from which to view previous descriptions of the relationship between movement parameters and resulting movement accuracy. Traditional accounts of the speed-accuracy function are shown to be either inaccurate or incomplete. Furthermore, previous postulates have failed to incorporate movement timing error, or, where it is a part of the speed-accuracy description (e.g., Schmidt, Zelaznik, Hawkins, Frank, and Quinn, 1979), the timing error function is independent of and incongruent with the spatial error function. The proposed space-time description provides an alternative perspective from which to assess the extant explanatory interpretations of the speed-accuracy phenomenon. These include information transmission (Fitts 1954), discrete error correction (Crossman and Goodeve 1963; Keele 1968), and motor-output variability (Schmidt, Zelaznik, and Frank 1978; Schmidt et al. 1979).

Movement Speed and Spatial Error

The speed-accuracy trade-off is the most reliable relationship in the movement control literature. Its essence is that spatial error, irrespective of the particular dependent variable, tends to increase with gain in movement velocity. Consequently, the principal tactic available to the performer to ameliorate such error is the reduction of movement speed so that, as the law implies, a trade-off is made between movement speed and resultant accuracy.

There have been many attempts to describe and to explain the speed-accuracy relationship. The major approaches are examined here in order to provide a basis for the proposed space-time description. At this juncture, focus is directed toward the various descriptive relationships that have been advanced between the kinematic variables and movement spatial-error, rather than the accompanying explanatory constructs. The individual accounts provide insight into restricted elements of the speed-accuracy function but none offers a comprehensive picture.

Woodworth. Woodworth (1899) in his dissertation research is often credited with being the first to examine the movement speed-accuracy relationship. However, an earlier treatise by Fullerton and Cattell (1892) on the psychophysics of movement preempts Woodworth's investigation and, in addition, references earlier experimental work by both German and French investigators on this problem. Although acknowledged as the seminal behavioral work in motor control, Woodworth's contribution might be viewed more veridically as a crystallization of the previous and somewhat sporadic research. Woodworth, working with his mentor Cattell, examined over 125,000 line drawing movements in an attempt to construct a cohesive account of the accuracy of voluntary movement. Despite the justifiable acclaim that Woodworth has received for this work, it is apparent that the rich description provided in his monograph of the interrelationship between movement time, distance, and velocity in the determination of movement error has been neglected.

It should be noted that in our projection of the Woodworth data, and all subsequent data sets, we examine the various response errors in relation to three movement parameters, namely, amplitude, movement time, and average movement velocity. Utilizing the redundant degree of freedom, average velocity, facilitates an intuitive understanding of the error functions and, in this first pass at synthesizing the speed-accuracy functions, we have kept average movement velocity in our graphical projections. Formal accounts of the speed-accuracy function should be able to accommodate the error function in terms of amplitude and time.

In experiments constructed to test the applicability of Weber's (1834) psychophysical theory to the movement domain, Woodworth independently manipulated 4 distances (5, 10, 15, and 20 cm) and 10 movement durations (300–3,000 ms) in a line drawing task. Only three subjects performed this experiment of which only one subject completed all conditions. The standard unit er-

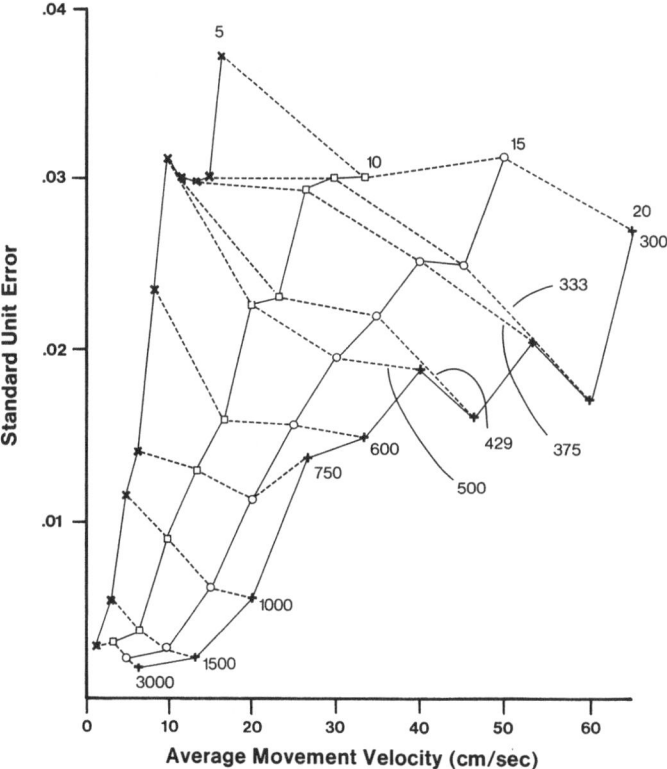

Fig. 1. Standard unit error as a function of average movement velocity. Within the body of the illustration movement times (*dotted lines*) extend from 300 to 3000 ms and movement amplitudes (*solid lines*) range from 5 to 20 cm in 5-cm increments. (Data redrawn from Woodworth 1899, Tables XVI–XVIII)

ror for each of the three subjects has been collapsed to form a group mean error for each time-distance combination and these means are depicted in Fig. 1.

As can be seen in the illustration we have had occasion to reference a newly labeled movement error called standard unit error which will recur throughout our treatise. This measurement is constructed from the within-subject standard deviation of response errors, commonly denoted as variable error (VE), together with the imposed spatial or temporal movement criteria. VE may be derived for both spatial and temporal aspects of response errors. The standard unit error for space represents the VE of amplitude divided by the imposed movement distance at which the error was observed. In essence, this form of error encapsulates the proportion of variable error made per imposed unit distance. In order that no misconception be formulated as to the dimension of this error, because it is dimensionless, we have referred to this as standard unit error. As we subsequently show, when standard unit error is calculated on the same principle for temporal error, these space-time aspects of movement error are homeomorphic in that they possess equivalent morphological features. The standard unit error is distinct from the coefficient of variation, for example, which divides the standard deviation of error by the attained mean, rather than the imposed mean as in the case of the present condition. Thus, the standard unit error is independent of constant error functions, which are subsequently developed in a separate section.

The decrease of standard unit error with increments of average velocity per given movement time indicates that the gains in variable error are not proportional to the distance moved, which would be consistent with Weber's theory, as error increases at a slower rate than changes in extent. However, the variable error increases at a faster rate than the square root of stimulus magnitude, a formulation originally postulated and tested by Fullerton and Cattell (1892). Woodworth's data also indicate degrees of alternating curvilinearity in the standard unit error at low- and high-velocity conditions within a single amplitude. Also, increases in movement time within a given distance reduce the standard unit error but by an amount less than would be proportional to the change in temporal duration.

Figure 1 clearly displays certain random trends particularly at the shortest movement times. This is presumably because some data points are based upon observations derived from a single subject. However, in contrast to the interpretation advanced by Keele (1968, p. 391), we choose to interpret the non-proportional and curvilinear trends exhibited in Woodworth's data as the basis for a veridical description of the speed-accuracy function.

Woodworth also reported systematic constant error shifts with changes in kinematics. The general trend within a given movement amplitude was for overshooting and undershooting to occur at low- and high-velocity conditions, respectively.

Woodworth's observations imply an intricate relationship between movement duration, amplitude, and velocity in the determination of movement error. However, this perspective has failed to emerge from subsequent reference to this work. This is surprising because Woodworth's dissertation still provides one of

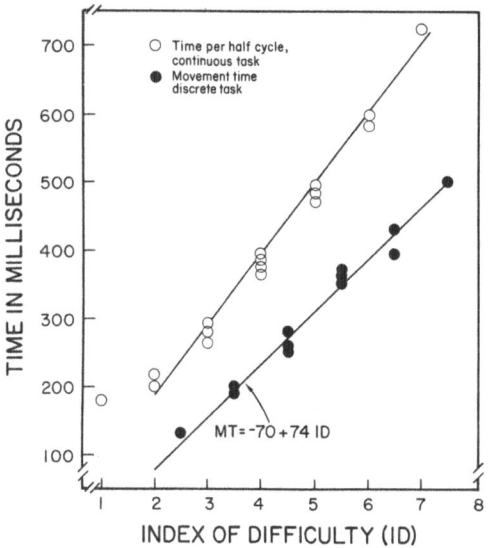

Fig. 2. Movement time (ms) as a function of index of difficulty (ID) in tapping (Fitts 1954) and discrete (Fitts and Peterson 1964) movement tasks. (Adapted from Fitts and Peterson 1964)

the most comprehensive investigations pertaining to the speed-accuracy relationship and, as we subsequently demonstrate, the data are consistent with more recent empirical observations (e.g., Schmidt et al. 1979).

Fitts. While Garrett (1922), Philip (1936), and Craik and Vince (1963a, b)[1] pursued descriptions of the speed-accuracy functions, it was Fitts (1954) who proposed a formal relationship:

$$MT = a + b \log_2 (2A/W). \tag{1}$$

where MT is movement time, A represents the amplitude of movement, W is the target width, and a and b are empirically determined constants. Data reflecting the accuracy of this mathematical relationship are shown in Fig. 2, which is taken from the discrete movement analysis of Fitts and Peterson (1964) and includes movement time data from the original tapping task protocol employed by Fitts (1954).

In Fitts' formulation, an index of movement difficulty (ID) is manipulated by the ratio of target width to amplitude of movement and is calculated by:

$$ID = \log_2 (2A/W). \tag{2}$$

Since Fitts' original proposal, several elaborations to Equation 1 have been advanced. Welford (1968) suggested that subjects utilize only the near half of the target area and modified the equation accordingly to accommodate a greater percentage of performance variance in the form:

$$MT = K \log_2 (A/W + 0.5). \tag{3}$$

---

[1] The original dates of these manuscripts were August, 1943 and March, 1944, respectively, published as APU reports, Cambridge University, England.

Subsequently, Welford, Norris, and Shock (1969) advanced an equation relating movement time separately to amplitude and target tolerance:

$$MT = a + b \log_2 A + b \log_2 (1/W). \tag{4}$$

Other investigators have followed Fullerton and Cattell (1892) and used the actual spatial error from a point or line target. These measures of error[2] of a distribution of trial responses have been labeled mean error square (E^2) and the effective target width (W_e), respectively (Beggs and Howarth 1970; Welford 1968). These procedures have allowed a more precise description of the distribution of the outcome of responses compared with a score of percentage of movements missed for any particular target width. However, these approaches do not preclude an error derived from the method of measurement employed. For example, Schmidt et al. (1978) estimated that with their procedure the measurement error of W_e in the stylus-aiming task was equal to 0.6 mm. The contribution of measurement error to the overall estimation of movement accuracy may be small, although it is still an important factor to consider in the full description of the speed-accuracy relationship.

The suggested modifications to Fitts' equation have added a marginal degree of precision to the quantification of the speed-accuracy formulation but they have not changed the essence of the relationship inherent in the original equation. Moreover, the relationship proposed by Fitts has been demonstrated as robust over a wide range of populations (e.g., Wade, Newell, and Wallace 1978; Wallace, Newell, and Wade 1978), with different anatomical units (e.g., Langolf, Chaffin, and Foulke 1976), in an underwater environment (e.g., Kerr 1973), and under microscopic conditions (e.g., Hancock, Langolf, and Clark 1973). It is only fitting, therefore, that Equation 1 is generally known as Fitts' law.

There are several factors indicating limitations to the potential of Fitts' law as a general description of the movement speed-accuracy relationship. With respect to its internal consistency, it has been observed that the lawful relationship fails at very low IDs (e.g., Crossman and Goodeve 1963; Klapp 1975), a feature illustrated in the original Fitts data (see the deviation from the regression line of the movement time for the tapping task at ID of 1 in Fig. 2). Secondly, in contrast to the implicit assumption of Fitts' law, it has been suggested that amplitude and target width do not possess equal weighting in the determination of movement time (Sheridan 1979). This criticism centers on the observation that in several aiming studies the movement times for amplitude-target combinations, within a particular ID, tend to be aligned in an inverse order with respect to target size so that smaller targets possess longer movement times. Unfortunately, it is uncertain whether this trend reflects departures from Fitts' law or experimental

---

[2] The confusion surrounding the use of the term "effective target width" has been compounded by different interpretations for this common label. Welford (1968), following Crossman (1957), took W_e to represent an error range represented by four standard deviations. Schmidt et al. (1979) utilized W_e as the within-subject standard deviation of response errors.

artifacts. For example, it is possible that this effect could be the result of a speed-accuracy trade-off within amplitude-target width conditions. However, this argument cannot be utilized with Fitts' (1954) original data as the smaller targets also possess the larger error rates.

A further possible confounding element is that larger targets increase the likelihood of a higher number of contacts occurring in the near half of the target. The outcome of such a constant error shift would be that the average distance traveled would decrease as target size increases at a given distance so that movement time also decreases proportionally for a given error rate. Consequently, there appear to be limitations in the Fitts formulation of the speed-accuracy function although problems with the aiming task protocol also compromise its internal validity.

In addition to the foregoing problems, the term speed when used in relation to Fitts' law has, in effect, assumed the burden of representing both a velocity and a time dimension as, in the Fitts discrete and reciprocal aiming tasks, the average movement velocity and movement time covary. The independent effects of movement amplitude, velocity, and duration on spatial accuracy were not presented by Fitts, or indeed in subsequent work concerning the Fitts protocol, although such relationships may be derived from Equation 1. Fig. 3 depicts the data originally presented in Fitts (1954, Experiment 1) but redrawn such that the relationships between movement time, amplitude, average velocity, and error (target tolerance) are explicit.

One striking relationship revealed in Fig. 3 is that error, as assessed by target tolerance, decreases in a curvilinear manner as average movement velocity decreases at any movement amplitude. If lines for prescribed movement times were drawn through the appropriate points of target tolerance, although this is not possible with Fitts' data set as there are no identical movement times despite the original prediction, then they would increase at a negatively accelerating rate

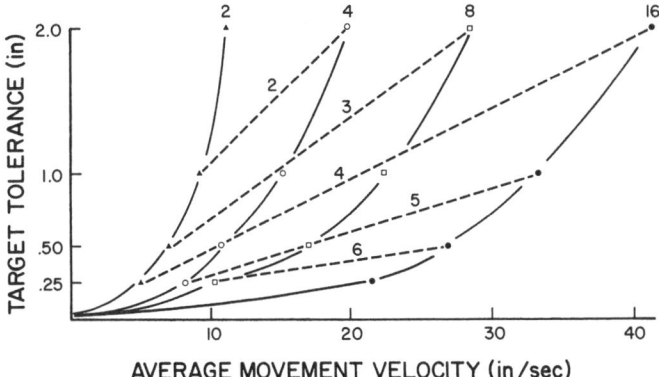

Fig. 3. Target tolerance (in.) as a function of average movement velocity (in./s), movement amplitude (in.) (continuous lines), and index of difficulty (*dashed lines*). (Redrawn from Fitts 1954, Table 1)

with gains in average movement velocity in a fashion consistent with the Wood-worth data previously reviewed. The *ID*-error (target tolerance) lines appear linear with a common intercept on the ordinate above the intersection of the axes. Our interpretation is that Fig. 3 is more revealing as an exposition of the basic relationships that exist between the kinematic parameters and movement error than was originally presented (see Fig. 2).

In addition to the above specific limitations, it is the case that all verifications of Fitts' law have occurred in aiming tasks with only one or two spatial criteria. There have been no attempts to determine whether Fitts' equation applies to a task with three measured spatial criteria. A more important restriction of the Fitts protocol is that movement time is a dependent rather than an independent variable and this excludes the concomitant consideration of temporal error to movement accuracy. This is a serious limitation particularly in considering tasks which have time as a criterion, as for example when a limb, or an extension of a limb, is required to make contact with a moving object.

Fitts' law also describes the movement speed-accuracy relationship princi-pally at the upper end of the movement velocity continuum for any particular anatomical unit over any given movement amplitude-target tolerance condition. It is only in limited circumstances that tasks demand limb movement at or ap-proaching that of maximum velocity for any particular movement amplitude. Even within this limited range of movement velocities, it has been suggested that the points utilized in the construction of the Fitts relationship may be more ap-propriately fitted to curves other than logarithmic transform (Jagacinski, Rep-perger, Ward, and Moran 1980; Kantowitz and Knight 1978). Indeed, Kvålseth (1980) has shown that a power function produces a marginally superior fit to data derived from Fitts' protocol, although only at the expense of adding an ad-ditional degree of freedom to the equation. Parenthetically, the base of the log component of Fitts' equation is immaterial to the description (Bainbridge and Sanders 1972). The binary base was chosen presumably to maintain a degree of concordance with the information theoretic approach of the original conceptions of Shannon and Weaver (1949), although the mathematical assumptions upon which such a connection to Fitts' formulation is founded have been suggested as flawed (Kvålseth 1979).

Given these reservations concerning Fitts' law, it seems necessary to consider the nature of the speed-accuracy relationship over a wider range of kinematic conditions and unbound by the particular constraints of the stylus-aiming pro-tocol. While Fitts' law provides a good approximation of the movement-speed spatial accuracy phenomenon, over a reasonably wide range of the movement velocity continuum, Equation 1 clearly cannot represent the comprehensive de-scription of it. Moreover, it masks certain systematic relationships that exist be-tween accuracy and the kinematic parameters of movement.

Finally, it should be recognized that it is important to distinguish between Fitts' equation as a description or curve-fitting operation of the relationship be-tween movement time and target tolerance and as an information transmission explanation which attempts to account for the speed-accuracy function. Regardless of the veracity of Fitts' law as a description it does not necessarily demand a tacit or explicit acceptance of the information transmission explanation by characterizing the relationship of *ID* to movement time in terms of channel capacity. There are grounds upon which to question the analogy drawn by Fitts between the information capacity of a band-limited communication channel and the human motor system. For example, Kvålseth (1979) has argued that in the classical model the input signals are stochastic whereas Fitts (1954) implied that the input to the motor system is deterministic. This latter assumption leads to fixed and consequently erroneous estimates of the information capacity of the human motor system. However, even with an appropriate use of communication theory, the derived channel capacity is merely an alternate form of description of the outcome variability for given kinematic conditions, in that it is obtained by rearranging the terms in Fitts' equation.

Bailey and Presgrave. In the course of developing principles and procedures relative to time and motion studies in the work place, Bailey and Presgrave (1958) conducted several analyses of the relationship between the speed and accuracy of simple limb movements. This work is not recognized generally in accounts of the movement speed-accuracy relationship, which is unfortunate as the data on the accuracy of simple arm movements represent one of the most comprehensive examinations conducted.

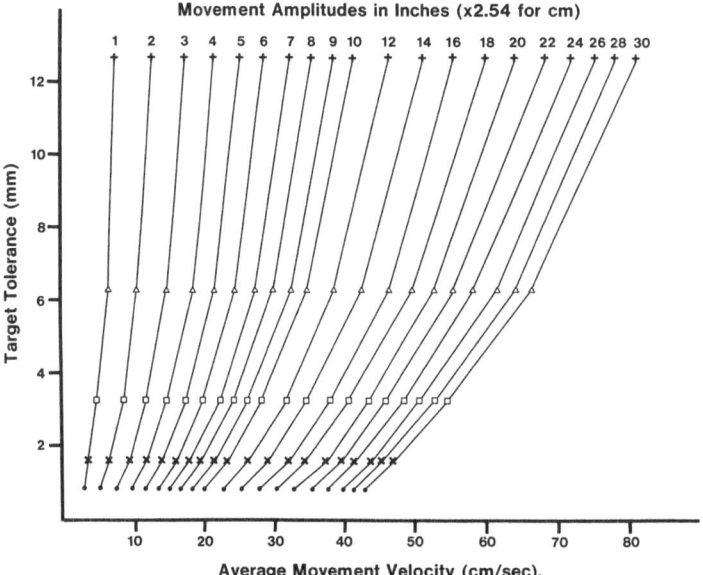

Fig. 4. Target tolerance (mm) as a function of average movement velocity (cm/s) and movement amplitude (in.). (Adapted from Bailey and Presgrave 1958; Figures 10, 13. The original scale for movement amplitudes is preserved for ease of illustration)

Figure 4 is adapted from data originally presented in Bailey and Presgrave (1958, Figures 10, 13) and describes the average velocities of arm movements to a target in terms of the 20 amplitudes and 5 target tolerances manipulated. Details of the experimental procedures are somewhat sparse but apparently there were no error rates as subjects were always required to contact the target regardless of temporal constraint. The data are consistent, however, in demonstrating the curvilinear relationship of movement velocity and target tolerance within a pre-scribed movement amplitude. In this respect the data of Bailey and Presgrave (1958) provide substantial support for the reinterpretation of the observations of Fitts (1954), which we have discussed above. Figure 4 also reveals that constant increments of amplitude at any given target tolerance lead to a negatively de-celerating increase in the average movement velocity produced. Consistent ef-fects are also noted for slope of the amplitude lines, which decrease systemati-cally with equal increments of movement amplitude.

In each case the data points presented are based on CV movements, those which Bailey and Presgrave note as requiring precision in movement (C) with the use of vision (V). From the current perspective one limiting factor of this work is the lack of specification of a defined temporal criterion. As a consequence, the picture presented in Fig. 4 may not be as veridical a representation as could be desired concerning the movement time contribution to overall accuracy.

Beggs and Howarth. On the basis of a series of hand-aiming experiments (Beggs and Howarth 1970, 1972 a, b), Howarth, Beggs, and Bowden (1971) determined that the mean square error (E^2) of the deviations from a target line was predicted by the equation:

$$E^2 = E_0^2 (o_\Theta d_u)^2. \tag{5}$$

where E_0 and o_Θ are empirically determined constants. Howarth et al. (1971) speculated that E^2 was made up of the sum of two independent sources of error. E_0^2 was taken to represent some kind of uncontrollable tremor while $(o_\Theta d_u)^2$ is a variance due to the angle (o_Θ) and length (d_u) respectively of what Howarth and colleagues referred to as the uncontrollable movement, which represents that portion of the movement produced by the last discrete error correction. It was determined that the aiming data revealed a linear relationship between mean square error (E^2) and the distance traveled during this last discrete correction.

Howarth et al. (1971) indicated that the speed-accuracy data generated from their experiments were incompatible with Fitts' formulation. However, there are several differences between the respective experimental protocols employed. The task utilized by Howarth et al. (1971) was distinct in that the aiming movement occurred in the sagittal plane, the duration of each tapping movement was rela-tively long (416–1428 ms) compared with that in Fitts' (1954) original work (180–731 ms), and the measures of spatial accuracy were orthogonal to the prin-cipal plane of motion. Kerr and Langolf (1977) have demonstrated that Fitts' law operates for movements in the sagittal plane and therefore the difference be-tween the formulation of Fitts and that of Beggs and Howarth is unlikely to be due simply to the influence of the selected plane of motion. Another possible source of incongruence is the difference in the duration of each individual movement. In the studies conducted by Beggs and Howarth, the movement times were considerably greater than those in Fitts' experiments and presumably allowed for a higher probability of discrete corrections over a group of trials.

Howarth et al. (1971), based upon earlier work (Beggs and Howarth 1970), fixed the temporal estimate of the last error correction from target impact at 290 ms. Consequently, the distance traveled during the last error correction covaried with the average velocity of the discrete correction. A reanalysis of the root mean square error (E) data reported by Howarth et al. (1971) reveals that E also increases as the average velocity of last discrete correction increases (see Fig. 5). Furthermore, when E is divided by the distance traveled during the proposed last error correction, the error decreases with increases in the average velocity of the corrective response (see Fig. 5). This implies that increases in E are not proportional to gains in both distance and velocity of the last discrete correction.

Discrete correction interpretations of Fitts' law (Crossman and Goodeve 1963; Keele 1968) operationally define a correction as an inflexion point on a trace of a kinematic parameter (e.g., Carlton 1979a, 1980; Langolf et al. 1976). Howarth and his associates did not measure the discrete movement corrections directly and in consequence their interpretation of the speed-accuracy relationship relies on the implication that a discrete correction occurred as the movement

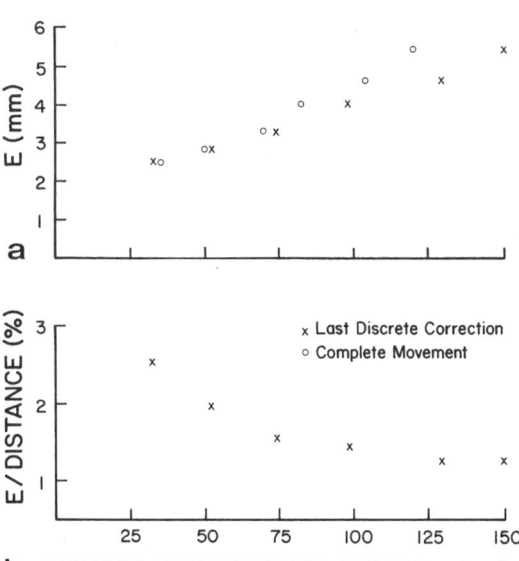

Fig. 5. a E, Root mean error square (mm) as a function of average movement velocity and average velocity of the final discrete correction. **b** E, divided by movement amplitude (%) as a function of the average velocity of the final discrete correction. (Adapted from Howarth, Beggs and Bowden 1971, Table 2)

times exceeded that of a visually based movement correction time. The temporal duration of a movement is insufficient a criterion from which to establish the presence or absence of a discrete correction.

Current estimates of the minimum visual processing time in discrete movements are considerably lower than the traditionally accepted 190–260 ms (Keele and Posner 1968) and 290 ms proposed by Beggs and Howarth (1970). Carlton (1981) utilizing high-speed film techniques has shown visually based discrete corrections with a latency of 135 ms, and Smith and Bowen (1980) have provided evidence that visually based response corrections can occur in less than 90 ms. Hence, even if discrete corrections occurred, the 290-ms estimate of minimal visual processing time by Beggs and Howarth is conservative. Indeed, Carlton (1979 b) has argued that perusal of the Beggs and Howarth (1970) data suggests that contrary to their own assessment the mean corrective reaction times were 165 ms when vision was withdrawn with the hand close to the target. The discrepant estimates apparently are due to the point in the movement trajectory where vision was withdrawn. When vision is withdrawn with the hand close to the target, Carlton proposes that the estimate of visual processing time is shorter than 290 ms and this estimate increases when the hand is farther from the target.

The summary kinematic data presented by Howarth et al. (1971, Figure 1) suggest that a continuous movement occurred on average although it is possible that these group data mask individual trial corrections which may have occurred. The failure to provide direct evidence of discrete corrections on individual trials undermines the interpretation offered by Beggs and Howarth for their speed-accuracy function. In addition, it raises the issue of whether the temporal duration of the response is the key factor which affords different functions for the speed-accuracy data sets presented by Fitts (1954), Beggs and Howarth (1970), and indeed, as will be subsequently discussed, Schmidt et al. (1979). Reanalysis of the data provided by Howarth et al. (1971) and Beggs, Graham, Monk, Shaw, and Howarth (1972) in terms of E divided by the amplitude of movement suggests that E increases nonproportionally regardless of whether it is related to the average velocity of the last discrete correction or the average velocity of each movement (see Fig. 5).

In summary, the formulation of Beggs and Howarth cannot represent a general account of the movement-speed accuracy relationship as it is limited to measurements of spatial error and constrained to movements that are assumed to contain a discrete correction. It is our contention that the actual data of Fitts and those of Beggs and Howarth are qualitatively similar and differ only quantitatively due to the differing task demands alluded to previously. In addition, apparent differences may be generated by the use of a logarithmic axis as is given in Howarth et al. (1971). The absolute size of the movement errors will inevitably be smaller when they are measured on the basis of aiming movements to a target line and in a plane orthogonal to the principal direction of motion, which probably renders the employment of Crossman's (1957) estimate of effective target width by Howarth et al. (1971) inappropriate for contrasting the data sets.

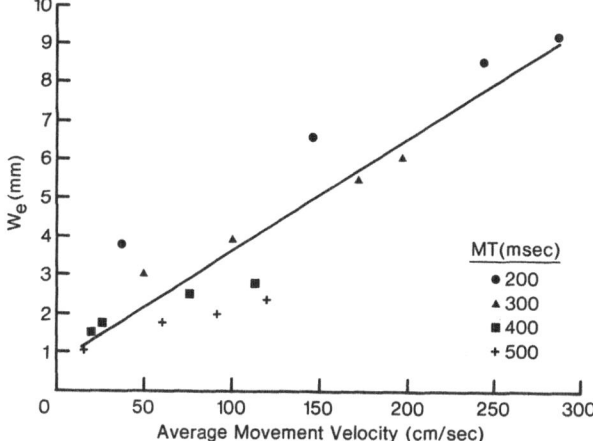

Fig. 6. Effective target width (W_e) or standard deviation of spatial error as a function of average movement velocity. (From "Motor output variability: A theory for the accuracy of rapid motor acts" by Schmidt, Zelaznik, Hawkins, Frank and Quinn, Psychological Review, 1979, *86*, 415–451, Figure 7. Copyright 1979 by the American Psychological Association. Adapted by permission of the publisher and author)

Schmidt, Zelaznik, Frank, Hawkins, and Quinn. In support of a motor-output variability theory of the movement speed-accuracy trade-off, Schmidt et al. (1978, 1979) have presented spatial-accuracy data for aiming movements, over a range of average movement velocities (15–300 cm/s) and movement times (140–500 ms). Figure 6, which is derived from Schmidt et al. (1979, Figure 7), provides their picture of movement spatial error in a two-dimensional aiming task. Schmidt et al. recognized two trends in the data depicted in Fig. 6: firstly, a linear relationship between average movement velocity and spatial error in the form of W_e, a finding which is consistent with Weber's law and, secondly, the tendency for both slope and intercept of the regression line on W_e to increase as movement time decreases. This suggests that movement time and average movement velocity interact in determining spatial error (W_e) measured in the principal direction of motion. Increases in movement velocity have been shown also to increase error in the plane orthogonal to the principal direction of motion (Begbie 1959; Beggs and Howarth 1970; Drury 1971), although the absolute size of error is reduced in this plane (Siddall, Holding, and Draper 1957; and compare Schmidt et al. 1979; Figures 8, 10).

A linear relationship between actual variable spatial error and movement velocity was reported by Schmidt et al. (1979) in the form:

$$W_e \propto (A/MT) \tag{6}$$

where A is movement amplitude and MT is movement time. However, there are reasons to doubt the validity of this description. If the relationship was linear, it would be in direct conflict with each of the preceding descriptions of the movement-speed spatial-accuracy phenomenon, including Fitts' formulation, which only appears linear by virtue of the logarithmic term in Equation 1. In addition, a proportional function is incongruent with the curvilinear relationship established between movement velocity and timing error (Newell et al. 1979, 1980). Consequently, there are grounds upon which to postulate that the spatial error movement-velocity relationship is not a simple linear function. A linear function between response variability and movement velocity for prescribed amplitudes was rejected by Fullerton and Cattell (1892) and Woodworth (1899) in their original investigations of Weber's law concerning movement precision.

Indeed we propose that a more veridical picture emerges from a reanalysis of the data of Schmidt et al. (1979) presented in Fig. 6. Although Schmidt and his colleagues interpreted the speed-accuracy function from their data as linear it is our contention that a curvilinear function is more appropriate. One problem encountered is that linear trends may often be fitted to a small number of data points and interpretation may be also biased by the relative scales chosen for use on ordinates and abscissae. Figure 7 reflects a reexamination of the actual values presented in Schmidt et al. (1979) and reveals the curvilinearity of the movement-speed, spatial-accuracy function.

Figure 7 shows some interesting trends relative to the movement speed-accuracy relationship. Firstly, the standard unit error actually *decreases* curvilinearly as movement velocity increases with a given movement time. This finding is consistent with the functions generated from Woodworth's data which were presented in Fig. 1. Secondly, decreasing movement time at any given average velocity generates a negatively accelerating increase in the standard unit error.

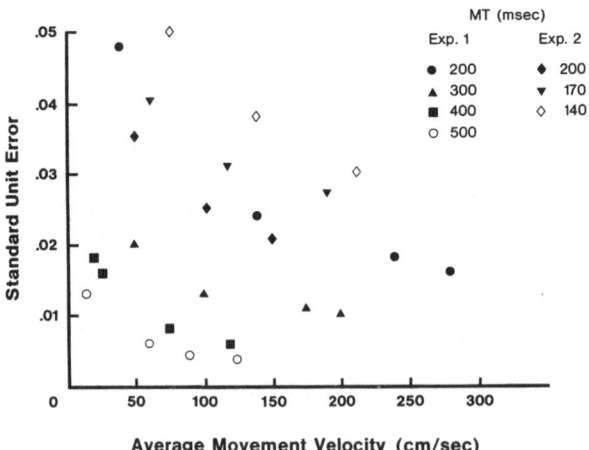

Fig. 7. Standard unit error as a function of average movement velocity and movement time. (From "Motor output variability: A theory for the accuracy of rapid motor acts" by Schmidt, Zelaznik, Hawkins, Frank, and Quinn, Psychological Review, 1979, *86*, 415–451, Figures 7, 9. Copyright 1979 by the American Psychological Association. Adapted by permission of the publisher and author)

This holds for movement times ranging from 140 to 500 ms in the data of Schmidt et al. and from 300 to 3,000 ms in the investigation of Woodworth. Thirdly, the rate of gain of error with decreases in movement time reduces at a negatively accelerating rate as distance increases. Thus, the trends exhibited in Fig. 7 show a remarkable degree of similarity to those depicted in Fig. 1 from Woodworth, despite the different task and time-distance constraints imposed.

We recognize the potential flaw in equating differing data sets on the graphical reinterpretation expressed in standard unit error terms. Indeed, various functions including both constant and straight-line relationships provide similar graphical morphologies when expressed in this manner. However, this only arises when the functions contain intercepts other than at the origin. We believe that when the subject engages in no movement, no error is made. Or in variable error terms the function tends toward zero as movement velocity decreases. As we have indicated earlier, this important tendency may be masked by measurement error. However, the passage of the variable error function through the origin makes the resulting expressions in standard unit error a veridical reflection of nonproportionality, rather than an artifact of dividing a straight-line function with an intercept by a constant.

The data presented by Schmidt and his colleagues provide interesting insights into the relationship between movement speed and accuracy, particularly with respect to isolating the impact of the various movement parameters upon the speed-accuracy phenomenon. However, Schmidt et al. (1979) failed to exploit fully the relationships indicated in their extensive data. Meyer, Smith, and Wright (1982) have utilized the empirical data provided by Schmidt and his colleagues and have claimed to provide a superior mathematical derivation of the linear trend noted. However, this model continues to adhere to a proportional interpretation of the relationship between the variability of error and movement velocity, a position which has been demonstrated to be essentially untenable.

Summary. It should be apparent from the preceding analysis that a comprehensive description of the movement speed-accuracy relationship has still to be realized. The existing accounts are either fundamentally incorrect or at best incomplete. Fitts' law has proved to be robust over numerous experimental conditions but does not account for the complete range of movement amplitude, time, and velocity manipulations and, indeed, has other limitations with regard to its potential as a general account of movement accuracy in three spatial dimensions with time as an added consideration. Furthermore, the speed-accuracy link between movements which are presumed to have (Howarth et al. 1971) and not have (Schmidt et al. 1979) a discrete correction prior to target impact is far from clear.

We now lay out a movement speed spatial-accuracy description which is based on the reinterpretations of the data sets previously presented together with other speed-accuracy analyses (e.g., Philip 1936). This description provides a basis for an understanding of the relative contribution of the various movement parameters to movement accuracy. Furthermore, this formulation is consonant with the movement-speed timing-error function, which is an essential precondition to the development of a space-time formulation of the speed-accuracy relationship.

The Movement-Velocity Spatial-Error Function

Initially it is necessary to consider the appropriate error measure(s) for depicting the movement speed-accuracy function. Most empirical examinations of this function have followed Fitts (1954) in utilizing a designated target width for aiming tasks. This is presumably, in part, for the purposes of ease of measurement and to preserve the theoretical link to Fitts' law. Although it has been suggested that estimates of W_e may be generated from this approach (e.g., Welford 1968), this proposal is dependent upon the assumption of normality of the response distribution across the target. An analysis of actual distributions belies this inference (Fullerton and Cattell 1892). It is appropriate, therefore, to measure the actual outcome obtained as precisely as possible in order that an accuracy representation may be generated of the total distribution of response outcomes at any given movement time-amplitude condition. This approach is consistent with the strategy initiated originally by Fullerton and Cattell (1892) and Woodworth (1899) to examine the speed–accuracy relationship.

The estimation of the distribution of response outcome errors for the speed-accuracy function is usually based upon two descriptive statistics, namely the mean and the standard deviation. In early investigations both statistics were reported separately (e.g., Fullerton and Cattell 1892; Woodworth 1899). In most subsequent investigations the performance mean or constant error either has not been provided (e.g., Schmidt et al. 1979) or it has been combined with variable error to form a root mean square measure (e.g., Howarth et al., 1971). One problem with omitting an independent assessment of mean performance from the speed–accuracy relationship is that the variability function is developed on the basis of the imposed amplitude-time constraints without consideration of the actual average velocity which is produced. The significance of imposed versus attained performance is particularly important at low and high average velocity conditions within any criterion amplitude, as constant spatial error shifts occur in the form of overshooting and undershooting, respectively (e.g., Fullerton and Cattell 1892; Woodworth 1899). Even if both the constant error and standard deviation functions are plotted there are additional features of the response error distribution which have not been considered in previous descriptions of the speed-accuracy function.

Accounts of the speed-accuracy function implicitly assume a normal distribution of response outcomes (e.g., Welford 1968). Consequently, descriptions of response outcome have been formulated upon only the first and second moments of a distribution. Skewness and kurtosis have not been considered, despite the fact that they may bias the estimates of the standard deviation if they are manipulated independently over a set of related distributions (Newell and Hancock 1984). Thus accounts of the speed-accuracy function have failed to consider the complete statistical properties of the response outcome distribution. This may be due in part to the misleading labels such as effective target width W_e (Schmidt et al. 1979), which are utilized for what in essence is simply the standard deviation of the response error.

The above statistical considerations have been raised as elaboration of the existing speed-accuracy accounts into a unified comprehensive function clearly depends upon an established and common set of descriptive statistical procedures. Furthermore, our interpretation is that discrepancies which occur between extant accounts are, in part, based upon statistical properties of distributions observed. Consequently, we begin our account of movement-speed and spatial accuracy by reference to the first distributional moment reflected in the functions for constant error (CE).

Fullerton and Cattell (1892, Figures 3, 4) demonstrated that constant error shifts occurred with changes in the amplitude of movement. However, Woodworth's experiments (1899, Tables XVI, XVIII) illustrate more systematic and revealing functions for constant error. As velocity demands increase within a given movement amplitude, the absolute value for constant error alters from a positive to a negative value. This connotes the change in tendency from spatial overshooting to undershooting as velocity increases. This is reflective in part of the range effect which occurs in the reproduction of amplitudes without time constraints (e.g., Brown, Knauft, and Rosenbaum 1958) and in the estimation of prescribed temporal intervals (Clausen 1950). Woodworth's data also show that the absolute size of constant error which occurs in undershooting is greater than in overshooting. Thus the effect noted for constant error does not appear symmetrical over the velocity continuum for any particular amplitude. Finally, Woodworth's experiments suggest that the zero crossing point for constant error occurs at approximately 50% of the maximum velocity for any prescribed amplitude.

Figure 8 depicts the proposed constant error function in the principal direction of motion for increases of average movement velocity, with four movement

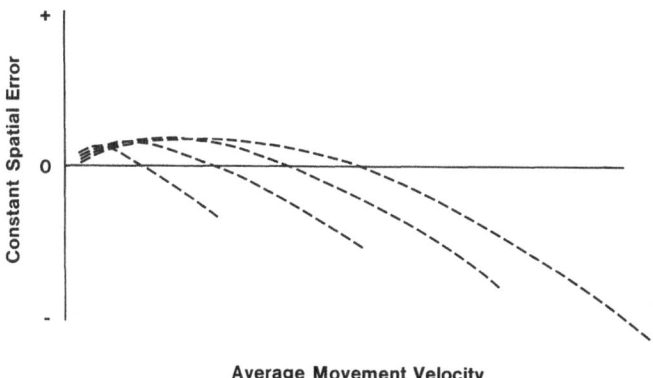

Average Movement Velocity

Fig. 8. Constant spatial error as a function of average movement velocity for equal increments of movement amplitude

amplitudes of equal increasing increments. Within each amplitude illustrated, positive constant error increases initially to be followed by an apparent peak which leads to a subsequent decrease up to approximately 50% of the maximum velocity. After crossing zero, constant error follows an increasing negative trend. However, in absolute terms the size of this negative constant error is increased and undershooting continues up to a maximum average velocity for any prescribed amplitude. The exact function for the asymmetry of under- and overshooting and the relative increment in constant error as a function of amplitude cannot be ascertained from existing data. For example, it is not certain whether the peak overshooting error increases with equal increments of movement amplitude. Nevertheless, the general function presented in Fig. 8 is consistent with the available constant error data given by Fullerton and Cattell (1892) and Woodworth (1899).

In practice it is expected that the proposed constant error functions are masked in the middle portion of the velocity range for a given movement amplitude. This is because measurement errors at these conditions are as large as average constant error which will tend in practice to distort estimates of the proposed function. This bias will be reduced at the extremes of the velocity range, particularly the high-velocity conditions, where, because of absolute size, constant error shifts are most easily observed (e.g., Woodworth 1899).

An appreciation of the constant error function is important as it indicates that the average *attained* response is not always equivalent to the *imposed* task conditions. Thus assessment of the response variability functions must be made in light of these constant error shifts. In the functions that follow we do not accommodate this problem directly by plotting the variability function on the basis of the attained average velocity. Rather, the obtained variability function is plotted on the basis of the imposed task velocity constraints to allow direct contrast with the attained constant error function illustrated in Fig. 8.

The proposed relationship between movement duration, amplitude, and standard unit error across the complete range of the movement velocity continuum is depicted in Fig. 9. The error function is for the standard unit error generated in the principal direction of motion for a discrete aiming task. A qualitative assessment is provided below concerning movement parameter–error relationships, which are shown within the boundary constraints of Fig. 9.

Figure 9 is constructed with the dashed lines representative of equal increments between movement amplitude and the continuous lines representative of equal increments between movement time. Three important and related aspects of the movement speed–accuracy relationship for variability are revealed. Firstly, within a given movement time, the standard unit error decreases at a negatively decelerating rate with constant increments in movement velocity. Secondly, within a given distance, the standard unit error increases in an ogival fashion with increments in average movement velocity. Thirdly, gains in standard unit error are not proportional to equal increments in either amplitude or time. Each of these general functions is now considered in some detail.

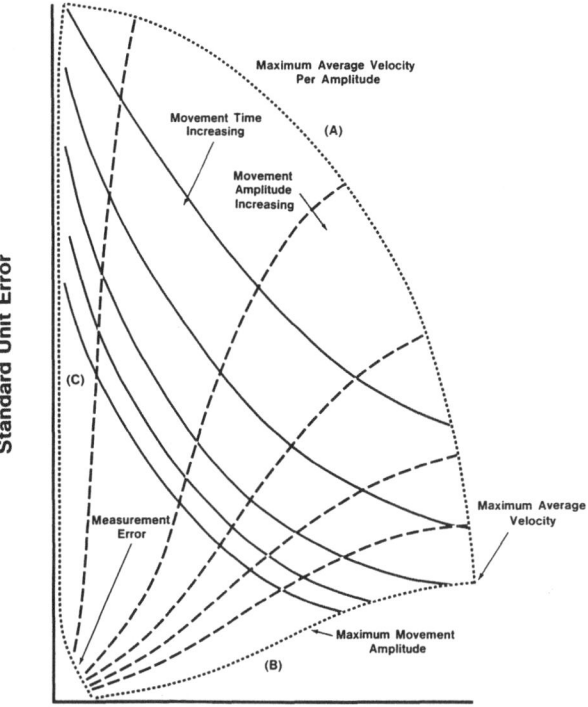

Average Movement Velocity

Fig. 9. Standard unit error as a function of average movement velocity, movement time, and movement amplitude. The error shown for movement amplitude (*dashed lines*) and movement time (*solid lines*) represents equal increments within each movement parameter. Physical, volitional, and measurement boundaries are represented by *dotted lines,* the description of which appear in the text

The reduction of the standard unit error with increments of movement velocity at a given movement time is consistent with the reinterpretation of the data of Woodworth (see Figure 1) and Schmidt et al. (see Figure 7). This relationship is apparently independent of feedback factors associated with time constraints, as the function is observed with movement times as short as 140 ms (Schmidt et al. 1979) and as long as 3,000 ms (Woodworth 1899). Thus response variability is not proportional to distance within a given movement time.

The ogival type error function for increments of movement velocity within a given distance has not been generally recognized. This is because most examinations of the speed-accuracy function have employed targets of a designated width and on those occasions where actual measurement error has been recorded the full velocity range has not been manipulated within a given distance.

Furthermore, as Philip (1936) has indicated, veridical estimates of error are difficult to determine at less than 10% and greater than 90% of maximum velocity. The ogival-type function indicates that the standard unit error for a given distance increases at an increasing rate to 50% of maximum velocity and then increases at a decreasing rate to maximum velocity. The curvilinear function at the lower end of the velocity continuum is consistent with the data sets of Woodworth (1899) and Schmidt et al. (1979) and also, in absolute values, with those using target tolerances (see the reinterpretation of Fitts' data in Figure 3 and the data of Bailey and Presgrave 1958, in their Figures 10 and 13). The data given by Woodworth (1899) confirm a curvilinear function at the upper end of the velocity continuum for any given amplitude.

Philip (1936) provided a clear demonstration of an ogival error function for increments of velocity in a stylus-aiming task. The task was different from Fitts' protocol in that subjects aimed a stylus at a hole inserted in a band of paper which was affixed to a drum rotating at varying velocities. As the velocity of the drum increased for a given preview amplitude the percentage of misses followed an ogival error function. Thus the complete function for standard unit error within a given distance is of an ogival morphology. It is unclear whether the amplitude function is symmetrical, as is the case with a true ogive, but there are no available data which contradict this supposition.

Increasing movement time at any given amplitude decreases the standard unit error in the form of a negative descending exponential. This implies that estimates of temporal duration in discrete aiming movements do not follow the proportional principles as given in Weber's law. An exponential function for timing variability as a function of temporal interval has been reported previously in time estimation studies (e.g., Michon 1967; Wing and Kristofferson 1973 a, b). It is important to note that increasing amplitude at a given movement time produces a similar standard unit error function.

Analysis of skewness and kurtosis of the response distribution lends coherence to the proposed interpretation of the constant error and standard deviation functions for movement speed-accuracy (Newell and Hancock 1984). Figure 10 shows the response distribution of error for a given amplitude over the range of achievable average movement velocities. The response distribution shifts from high leptokurticness and a modicum of positive skewness at low velocity through a normal distribution at 50% average velocity to high negative skewness and a modicum of platykurticness at high average velocity (Fullerton and Cattell 1892). Changes in either skewness or kurtosis do not *cause* changes in the standard unit error function of the response error, although they may influence the second moment (or its variants) in particular circumstances (Newell and Hancock 1984). Rather, an understanding of how all four moments vary with the kinematic conditions is required to depict fully the speed-accuracy function. In principle, N moments of a distribution can be calculated but in practice moments beyond the fourth power tend to be unstable (Hoel 1971).

Given the deviation from normality of the error distribution illustrated in Fig. 10, it is apparent that discussion of the standard unit error or any variability statistic of error cannot be undertaken meaningfully without reference to concomitant variations in the third and fourth moments or indeed the first moment.

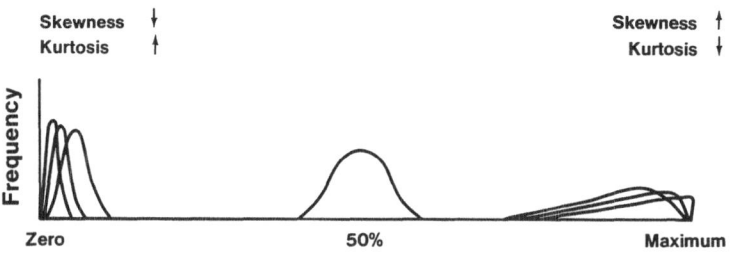

Average Movement Velocity

Fig. 10. Frequency distributions, each with an equal number of observations, for conditions at a constant movement amplitude throughout the average movement velocity continuum. Deviations of skewness and kurtosis are presented and detailed in the text

Thus changes in kinematic constraints produce variations in response error which are not captured sufficiently by assessment of the mean and standard deviation. As an example, the ogival type function for standard unit error for velocity increments within a given amplitude holds a different significance if the distributions are normal than if they are skewed and peaked. We cannot ascertain the relative contribution of shifts in the third and fourth moments and changes in variability per se to the ogival function for standard unit error. Consequently, in order to describe adequately differing distributions, the four descriptive statistics are at least necessary. This is particularly significant in examining inferences from distributions of response errors generated over the movement-velocity continuum.

Within the body of Fig. 9 the movement amplitude and time lines exhibit systematic changes in slope as both amplitude and time increase. A graphic example of this sequential change in slope is particularly obvious in the data of Bailey and Presgrave (1958) as given in Fig. 4. As may be seen the slope of the lines for amplitude decreases with equal increments across the range of values shown. In addition, the separation between the lines of amplitude also decreases as the absolute value ascends. In the illustration from the work of Bailey and Presgrave, there is an interruption in this smooth incrementation where amplitude change increases from 1 in. (2.54 cm) to 2 in. (5.08 cm) at the 10 in. (25.4 cm) value (see Fig. 4). These regularities for both slope and separation between increments of lines of amplitude are also true for the lines of movement time as shown for empirical data in Figs. 1 and 7 and for our idealized version in Fig. 9.

We have attempted to plot such regularities and specifically have taken values for the slope of amplitude and time lines as shown in the data set of Schmidt and his colleagues (Fig. 6). These data form what have been labeled K functions, which relate the veridical value of each slope with the amplitude or time from which it was derived. In calculating the respective K functions for amplitude and time we have as noted taken advantage of the absolute values reported in the extensive data set of Schmidt and his colleagues, although these may have equally as well been generated from the values reported by Woodworth (1899) as shown in Fig. 1. The subsequent K functions as given in Fig. 11 illustrate that for variable error, slopes of both movement amplitude and movement time decrease as both time and amplitude increase. If, as is possible, these K functions were generated for amplitude and time in standard unit error, rather than variable error as illustrated, then slopes for the amplitude lines should remain positive while slopes for the movement time would be negative. This latter observation indicates the juxtaposed nature of amplitude and time lines in standard unit error (see Fig. 9). However, it does not disturb the homeomorphic nature of the space-time picture. Although the ordinates have not been equated (except for illustrative purpose) the similarity of morphology is suggestive of an equal incrementation between values of time and amplitude within the constraints of the data produced by Schmidt et al. (1979).

To appreciate the limits of the relationship proposed in Fig. 9, it is useful to explore the various boundary conditions that may be assumed to exist. The distribution of errors at small amplitudes may not include the case where a trial or trials are generated in a direction diametrically opposed to the criterion direction of motion. In this situation, subjects are failing to achieve the objective of the task in a qualitative rather than quantitative manner.

There is a maximum average velocity which may be generated at any given movement amplitude. Fullerton and Cattell (1892, p. 115) demonstrated that the minimum time to move through ascending amplitudes (10–70 cm) increases at a

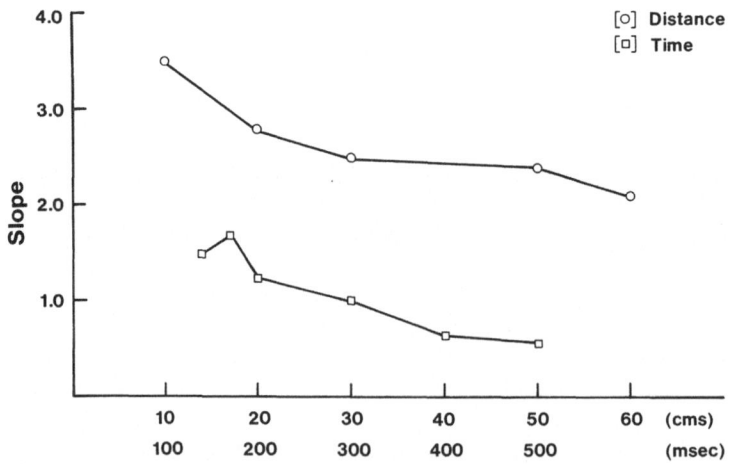

Fig. 11. The K functions (change of slope) for distance and movement time. One coincident point in the movement time function has been exempted from the construction of the respective K functions. (From "Motor output variability: A theory for the accuracy of rapid motor acts" by Schmidt, Zelaznik, Hawkins, Frank, and Quinn, Psychological Review, 1979, *86*, 415–451, Figures 7, 9. Copyright 1979 by the American Psychological Association. Adapted by permission of the publisher and author)

decreasing rate. Wadman, Denier van der Gon, Geuze, and Mol (1979, Figure 3) indicated that over a limited range (6–32 cm), this relationship was essentially linear, although an analysis of their slope and intercept indicates that such a function is most probably curvilinear toward the origin at decreased movement amplitudes. These studies have examined a limited range of conditions concerning the maximum average velocity–movement amplitude relationship.

In a recent experiment, we (Newell, Hancock, and Robertson, 1984) have examined minimum movement times to traverse ranges of motion from 2½% to 100% in an elbow flexion task. Results indicated that the maximum average velocity increased at a negatively accelerating rate with increments of distance up to 95% of the range of motion and this velocity limitation is reflected by Line A in Fig. 9. This function suggests an additional physical boundary. There is a limitation on the maximum average movement velocity that may be generated which occurs at the intersection of Line A with the amplitude constraint dependent on the length of the limb(s) utilized for activity (Line B). The functional limit to the present relationship is probably dependent upon anatomical and morphological constraints imposed upon the limb(s) used for movement. In practical terms this boundary may be in part dictated by the constraints of the task at hand.

The above boundaries are determined by the task constraints and the physical capabilities of the human system while the final limitation (Fig. 9, Line C) is related to the precision of the recording method(s). This boundary to the observable movement-velocity spatial error function represents measurement error. Although this is consistent across differing amplitude and time conditions it is reflected by the curvilinear function C in Fig. 9 due to the nature of the measure of standard unit error. As previously noted, Schmidt et al. (1978), without stating their precise method of assessment, estimated measurement error as approximately 0.6 mm. Although relatively small, such error is important as it aids in masking the curvilinear nature of the contribution of varying movement amplitudes as movement velocity decreases toward the origin.

To summarize, Figs. 8–11 represent our interpretation of the movement-velocity spatial-error relationship. They have been developed from existing data for simple hand-aiming tasks. Some of the details of the function for each moment remain to be determined and others remain to be verified. Nevertheless, the functions developed represent a coherent framework which is consistent with the data sets available including recent empirical findings (cf., Wright and Meyer 1983).

The speed-accuracy functions represent statistical manifestations of the movement outcome for a range of movement amplitude-time combinations. The functions demonstrate that movement accuracy must be considered on the basis of the error distributions for the first four moments of each amplitude-time combination, rather than reliance on any single descriptive statistic. Furthermore, the functions provide a basis for the prediction of movement error based upon the estimate of minimal movement time for the amplitude traversed under a given set of task constraints. This is possible because the estimate of minimal movement time across the range of amplitudes represents the 100% maximal average velocity boundary. It is anticipated that the functions hold for all tasks although the absolute level of movement error will vary with the task constraints.

The shifts in error on a proportional basis are small for any single descriptive statistic. For example, the standard unit errors from Woodworth (1899) and Schmidt et al. (1979) indicate that although the shifts are consistent across amplitude-time conditions the change is within a bandwidth of 5% of the given amplitude. These small changes have been masked in previous accounts because only a limited range of the speed-accuracy function has been considered and the general reliance on absolute measures of response accuracy rather than relative measures.

Although the function for standard unit error is proposed as being consistent across differing practice conditions, the precise relationship between the movement parameters and the absolute size of error may change. Woodworth (1899) noted that as any performer approaches his maximum speed or accuracy for any task individual trials agree more and more closely, this being a phenomenon of practice curves. He also stated that should a point be reached at which trials were quite unvarying the absolute limit for that mode of particular task performance would have been reached. The nature of the internal relationship between the various movement parameters and how they contribute to standard unit error will depend not only upon elements of practice but also upon the intrinsic space-time bias of any individual task undertaken.

In accordance with previous findings (e.g., Begbie 1959; Beggs and Howarth 1970; Drury 1971) it is proposed that the movement-velocity spatial-error functions will also apply to error generated in planes orthogonal to the principal direction of motion, although the absolute size of such error will be considerably diminished. We recognize that the measurement of spatial error in three dimensions holds certain intrinsic problems. However, these specific problems are not elaborated in the present chapter. There is no evidence available to indicate what the function may be for tasks requiring radically different response dynamics but there are, at present, no fundamental objections to the assertion that they will follow the general relationships exhibited.

Attempts at relating spatial and temporal errors have been limited (Howells, Knight Weiss, and Kak 1979; Newell 1980) partly because of the confinement of studies to the original Fitts paradigm, where movement time is not an independent variable. However, there have been descriptions of timing error as a function of movement velocity (e.g., Newell et al. 1979, 1980) and these are now discussed as a precursor to the development of a movement speed timing-error function and subsequently the space-time account of movement speed-accuracy.

Movement Speed and Timing Error

Movements may be constrained solely by spatial criteria but this cannot be the case with time, as movement tasks always have spatial boundaries. Nevertheless, certain tasks have time as a criterion in the sense of moving through a prescribed amplitude or arriving at a precise location in a criterion movement time. Timing tasks have been employed to examine various theoretical issues in motor learning (e.g., Ellis, Schmidt, and Wade 1968; Newell 1974), but it is only recently that descriptions have been developed of a unidimensional movement-speed timing-accuracy relationship (Newell et al. 1979, 1980, 1982).

A consistent finding in discrete timing responses is that the shorter the movement time the smaller the timing error (Newell 1976; Schmidt 1969). Timing error is the difference between the criterion movement time and the obtained movement time for traversing a given amplitude. This may be the result of a range effect, as with greater movement time more time is available for the response to vary. Indeed, time-estimation studies involving simply key press responses suggest that such a range effect may be a contributor to error in temporal estimation (e.g., Woodrow 1951).

A problem with most extant movement timing studies is that the independent variables of duration and velocity have been confounded (e.g., Ellis 1969). Rarely has movement time been manipulated independently of average movement velocity. Consequently, it is commonly the case that high-velocity movements have short durations and low-velocity movements have long durations. The data from early studies which systematically varied movement time and velocity suggested that movement velocity may affect timing accuracy (Ellis et al. 1968; Schmidt and Russell 1972), although little was made at that time of these statistically nonsignificant effects.

In our laboratory we have developed a description of the movement-speed timing-accuracy relationship (Newell 1980; Newell et al. 1979; Newell, Carlton,

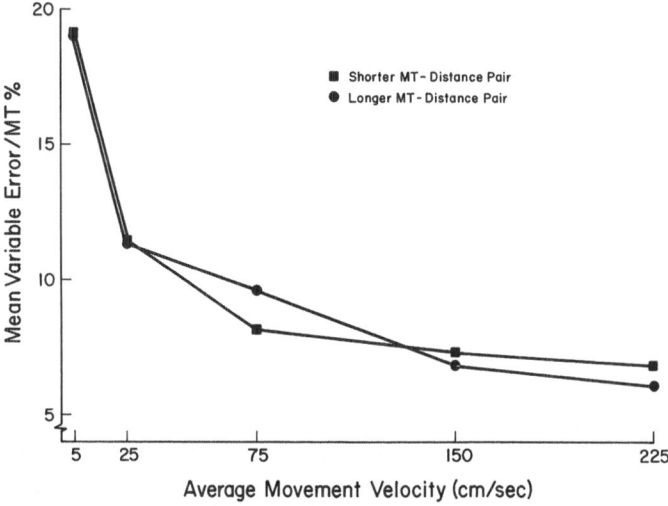

Fig. 12. Mean variability error movement time percentage (analogous to standard unit error) as a function of average movement velocity. (From Newell, Carlton, Carlton, and Halbert 1980, Experiment 3)

and Carlton 1982). At low velocities within a given distance subjects move too quickly and undershoot the temporal criterion whereas at high velocities they move too slowly and overshoot the criterion (e.g., Newell et al. 1980, Tables 2, 3). The constant timing error function is the complement of the constant spatial error function.

Figure 12 is adapted from Newell et al. (1980, Experiment 3) and reflects the movement-speed timing-accuracy function over movement velocities which range from 5 to 225 cm/s. The variable timing error is plotted as a percentage of movement time (standard unit error) in order to compare directly the timing error adduced from different movement times (100–600 ms). As Fig. 12 illustrates standard unit error decreases curvilinearly as a function of the average velocity of the discrete response. In Fig. 12 there is little or no difference for the standard unit error between different movement times at the same average velocity, but a graded movement time effect on the standard unit error has been shown with the proportionality of error to movement time decreasing as the duration of the response increased (Newell 1980; Newell et al. 1980, Figure 3). Timing error data consistent with this velocity function have also been reported by Sherwood and Schmidt (1980) and Tyldesly (1980).

In summary, the relative movement-speed timing error function appears to be homeomorphic with the spatial-error function. This is particularly clear in unidimensional tasks as the timing error may be directly reinterpreted in terms of concomitant spatial error (Newell et al. 1982) but the function also holds for timing error measured in a stylus-aiming task (Newell 1980). There are only a few data sets available to support the general timing error function which is presented in the following section. Nevertheless, the synthesis given above reflects a coherent description and one that is consistent with the spatial-error formulation presented previously.

The Movement-Velocity Temporal-Error Function

The work presented in the previous section together with that of the earlier projections of the standard unit error indicates that when temporal and spatial error are measured in the same movement plane, the error functions are homeomorphic. To facilitate contrast with the constant spatial error and standard unit error functions presented in Figs. 8 and 9, the constant temporal error and associated standard unit error functions will be shown separately.

The constant temporal error function is depicted in Fig. 13. Within a given amplitude, the constant temporal error increases from zero to a modicum of undershooting at low velocities, through zero constant error at approximately 50% of maximum velocity to a high degree of overshooting at high velocities. The constant temporal error function is in effect the complement of the constant spatial error function (cf., Figs. 8 and 13) in that movements are completed in a time shorter than the respective criterion at low velocities, with the reverse occurring at high velocities. Again, the constant error shift is not symmetrical around the 50% of maximum velocity for any given distance.

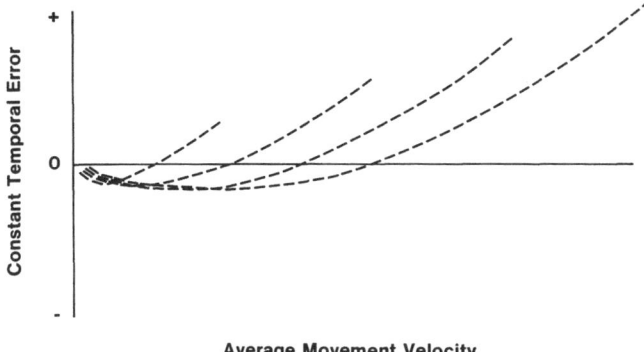

Fig. 13. Constant temporal error as a function of average movement velocity, for equal increments of movement time

The standard unit error function for time appears equivalent to the standard unit error function for space. It is probable that the actual proportions for these errors may differ but their form will be homeomorphic. Therefore, the standard unit error function for space, depicted in Fig. 9, also represents that for time. The standard unit error for time is generally about 5%–15% of the response duration whereas the standard unit error for space is between 0% and 5% of the amplitude moved. As shown previously in Fig. 11, the slopes of the standard unit error lines for amplitude and movement time (K functions) are in consonance with the homeomorphic interpretation of the independent space and time functions. It is worth noting that, unlike spatial error, timing error for a given movement time decreases with gains in movement velocity regardless of whether error is measured on a relative or absolute basis. This is because variable timing error is considered in relation to the same movement time over changing velocities whereas variable spatial error is considered over differing distances.

The response distributions for temporal error will also complement those for spatial error (Fig. 10). High negative skewness and a modicum of platykurticness will occur at lower velocities for a given distance and high leptokurticness and a modicum of positive skewness will result at the upper end of the velocity continuum. This bias in the third and fourth moments of the temporal error distributions for a given amplitude is shown in Fig. 14. Again the distributions are the complement of the respective spatial error distribution depicted in Fig. 10.

When timing error is measured in a plane orthogonal to that employed for spatial error the two functions may not be directly equated. The relationships expressed in Fig. 9 may be consistent for both temporal and spatial functions; however, the absolute size of error will vary in accordance with the plane of measurement (e.g., Begbie 1959). For example, in the Fitts tapping task, movement time is measured by contacting the horizontal plane, while spatial error is determined by the distance from the vertical plane placed through the target, with which contact is subsequently made. Hence, in studies which utilize Fitts' protocol the

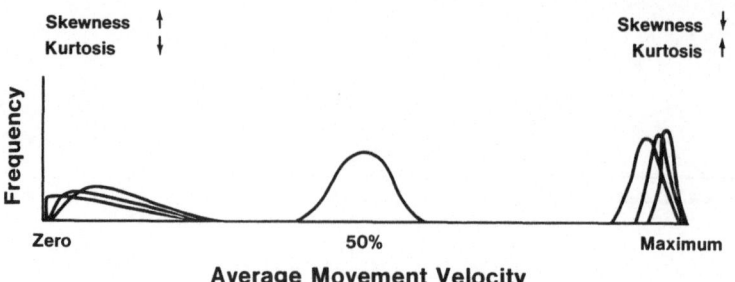

Fig. 14. Frequency distributions, each with an equal number of observations, for conditions at a constant movement time throughout the average movement velocity continuum. Deviations of skewness and kurtosis are presented and detailed in the text

movement time and spatial error functions are determined by cutting differing planes of motion.

In addition, the constraints of the Fitts stylus-aiming task dictate that there is a minimum movement time for the task which is considerably longer than both the interval scale of most time-keeping instruments and zero time. This is because a certain finite time is taken to raise and lower the stylus irrespective of the distance traveled in the principal direction of motion. Hence, the movement speed-accuracy function does not pass through the origin for the Fitts' stylus task (Crossman and Goodeve 1963; Fitts 1954; Fitts and Peterson 1964). Our speed-accuracy functions have been developed on the basis that graded movement times from zero time can occur on a very small interval scale and thus the functions (e.g., Fig. 9) tend toward the origin.

It is significant to note that in tasks with both space and time as criteria one cannot trade speed for accuracy in the traditional sense. We have indicated that one may trade spatial error for timing error but as these are different descriptions of the same event a trade, in the traditional sense, is untenable. Only where spatial and temporal errors are measured with reference to differing planes can a trade of spatial and temporal error occur. Again, Fitts' protocol may be viewed as creating a somewhat artificial condition for a movement trade-off in this case. This is not particularly useful if both space and time are criteria, although much depends upon the constraints of the task under consideration.

The independent development of the spatial and temporal error functions demonstrate that when both space and time are criteria for a task only a comprehensive space-time description of movement velocity–accuracy relationships is sufficient. The spatial and temporal error functions are homeomorphic, providing a unitary description and suggesting a common ground for explanation. To our knowledge there have been no attempts to describe movement–speed accuracy relationship in these terms.

It should be recognized that the space-time functions proposed reflect the movement outcome that *typically* occurs due to the constraints imposed in speed-accuracy studies. Changing the constraints on the subject in a movement accuracy task could alter the resultant movement speed-accuracy functions. Thus there is not a single space-time error function but rather a limited range of space-time functions according to task constraints (Newell, Carlton, and Hancock 1984). We now elaborate on the space-time perspective.

Movement Accuracy and Space-Time Considerations

The distinction between space and time as disparate entities may be perhaps simply a function of essential human experience. In scientific endeavour, the artificiality of this division has long been acknowledged. Locke (1690) commented upon the interdependency when he observed that expansion and duration mutually embrace and comprehend each other, where every part of space was in every part of duration. This position is in contrast to Newton's conception of time as a homogeneous medium in which events occur. Bergson (1910) criticized Newton's conception on philosophical grounds and suggested that time is event related. Subsequently, physicists have demonstrated the observer dependence of event order when events occur at highly disparate spatial locations. Minkowski (1908) in advocating the concept of space-time through the proposal of "world-points" enquired whether anybody had ever noticed a place except at a time or a time except at a place. In fact such was the mutual interdependency that Minkowski proposed the complete elimination of the concepts of space and time, leaving only "space-time."

It is axiomatic that movements which are generated to engage in action occur within this referential frame. However, as human action occurs essentially within a highly restricted spatial range, events *appear* upon a human scale as observer independent. As a consequence and in spite of both philosophical and physical developments, the Newtonian concept of time as absolute and measurable in a systematic manner has been and still is used in the motor control domain and in psychological investigation in general. Our current treatise has taken studies which have used the Newtonian referential frame and has constructed a space-time description account therefrom. However, we are aware that this space-time description differs from that in which Lee (1980) has observers navigate through the "world" (after Minkowski). It is conceivable that a space-time account of movement accuracy in the latter sense of the concept may emerge from the current work, which extracts information from accounts where the spatial and temporal contributions to movement accuracy are viewed as separate entities.

From the Newtonian perspective, it is clear that in many actions a movement or sequence of movements may be constrained to adhere to some greater or lesser degree to either spatial or temporal criteria. In the motor learning domain this is most evident in open skills where environmental contingencies are not entirely predictable between successive trials (Poulton 1957). The preceding discussion, which independently formulated space and time speed-accuracy functions, provides precursory arguments for the development of a space-time description of movement accuracy. In addition, it should be apparent that a space-time account is particularly appropriate where time is a set criterion of the performance rather than a dependent variable.

The unity of the space and time functions depends to a certain extent upon the technique employed to measure each dependent variable. When the errors are measured in relation to the same point in space and on the basis of movement in the same plane then the space and time error functions are homeomorphic. An example of this situation was demonstrated by Newell et al. (1982) when timing errors were determined for a variety of movement time-amplitude combinations on the basis of the difference from the criterion time on passing a point on a trackway, whereas spatial errors were determined by the distance from the target point at the criterion time. When the subject crosses the criterion spatial location earlier than the criterion movement time and decelerates after crossing the spatial target, departures from the homeomorphic nature of the spatial and temporal error functions may occur. However, for most movement conditions the spatial and temporal errors when measured in this manner will be homeomorphic as shown in Fig. 15A and B. In Fig. 15C and D the same recording technique was utilized but now subjects have different amounts of preload on the arm but attempt to travel the same distance in the same time (Carlton and Newell 1985). The standard unit error for the spatial and temporal functions is homeomorphic, reflecting the proposed space-time account of movement accuracy.

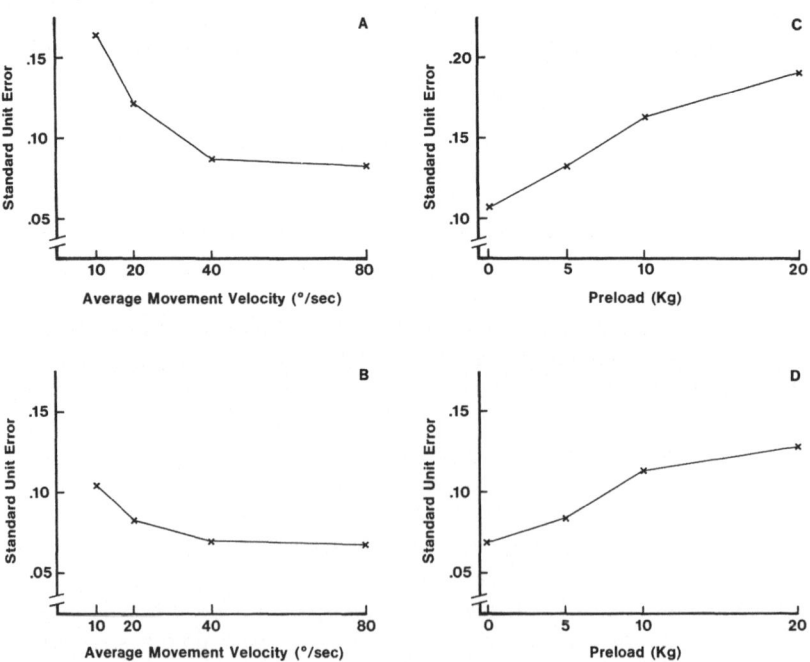

Fig. 15A–D. Standard unit error derived from timing error scores **A** and spatial error scores **B** adapted from Newell et al. (1982). **C** and **D** are standard unit errors derived from timing and spatial error scores of Carlton and Newell (1985)

In summary, the movement speed–accuracy relationship is a space-time problem. Emphasis may be placed upon the spatial or temporal consideration in training procedures but understanding the entire problem requires a merging of spatial and temporal measures into a space-time solution of the movement speed–accuracy relationship. Such an approach is not unique to the domain of movement.

Lee (1980) has recently proposed a space-time orientation in relation to the general problem of visual-motor coordination and specifically the nature of the information which is visually assimilated by the performer when interacting with the environment. As a result, Lee has developed a formerly dimensionless variable τ which affords information for controlling space-time activity. Finally, from an observer-independent perspective, Viviani and Terzuolo (1980) have demonstrated the principle of an invariant space-time domain in skills such as cursive handwriting and typewriting. In these skills the space-time topology is preserved independent of the absolute level of scaling observed in the spatial and temporal scales.

Implications of the Space-Time Description for Motor Control

In this treatise we have provided a coherent description of the speed-accuracy relationship in movement control. In order to promulgate such cohesion we have adopted a space-time perspective from which to approach the problem. This space-time approach is predicated on the notion that individual consideration of space and time artificially dichotomizes the phenomenon.

When space-time measures are considered in a single plane of motion their functions for variability are homeomorphic and the functions for the primary measure of central tendency, namely the distributional mean, are reflective images. Consequently space and time are not disparate entities but rather are direct reflections of each other in discrete movements. We point to Fitts' reciprocal tapping protocol as responsible for obfuscating this observation as errors of space and time in this approach, when measured, are for different movement planes.

An immediate ramification of our approach is that in space-time tasks one may not trade speed for accuracy; rather one may only trade spatial and temporal error and often this trade is dictated by the nature of the task under consideration. While most tasks have spatial criteria, fewer exhibit necessary temporal criteria. However, this does not make the latter any the less space-time tasks, it merely highlights one criterion in juxtaposition with the other.

In formulating the space-time approach it was observed that previous constructs were based upon limited consideration of the distribution of responses in demand to kinematic impositions. In our work we have suggested that in addition to distinct consideration of both the mean (central tendency) and standard deviation (variability), higher distributional moments must be considered as they are positive and implicit in distributions. Particularly they are noticeable at the extremes of movement capability (i.e., maximum and minimum velocity for any amplitude). Such considerations are necessary to understand the homeomorphic space-time function for movement variability at differing kinematic coordinates.

The cohesion of the current account and its contrast with previous, limited descriptions implies important failures in former theoretical accounts of the phenomenon at hand. We suggest, not only do these constructs fail quantitatively as they have accounted for only segments of the movement-speed trade-off, but also qualitatively in that they fail to meet the self-imposed criteria for causality in theoretical development. The appeals to lower levels of analysis for explanatory power have largely confused rather than facilitated further development. We do not feel it incumbent upon us to produce a similar and poorly founded theoretical position. Rather, we would care to make clear the importance of the current description.

First, there is a strong, although not causal, link between the kinematics and kinetics of movement, as Newtonian mechanics dictates. This position, previously advocated by Schmidt et al. (1979), implies principled relationships between kinematic and kinetic parameters of movement. However, unlike Schmidt and his colleagues we do not wish to suggest that this is causal in nature. The space-time description herein contained facilitates the development of understanding such connections and is the subject of current research efforts (Newell, Carlton, and Hancock, 1984; Schmidt and Sherwood 1982). Second, although our description militates against an iterative feedback model, and in this we are not the first (Legge and Barber 1976), we do envisage a role for feedback in movement control. However, our central concern is that such a process is not *manifest* in our description due to the distributional nature of the error measure. We believe the multiple-trial approach masks modes of control by a process of trial averaging. It is these specific elements of control that a *causal* theory would wish to address. In consequence, a single-trial analysis is advocated as one which, if receiving more attention, may be used to approach such problems.

Furthermore, although single-trial analysis may elucidate certain control processes, ongoing strategies for minimizing variation in performance should be addressed by some form of time-series examination. Our description suggests that the output of the motor system, in response to kinematic criteria, is a parametric production which is modified in consideration of physical limitations. That such output occurs suggests some form of sequential selection of response and those processes which produce such a response are those which it is necessary for future research to address.

Acknowledgments. This research was supported in part by the National Science Foundation under Award Number DAR 80-16287 and by an NIH Senior Fellowship, both to K. M. Newell. We would like to thank David Berg for his valuable input with respect to the development of the space-time description and Les Carlton, Herbert Heuer, Richard Jagacinski, Richard Schmidt, George Stelmach, and two anonymous reviewers for their helpful comments on an earlier version of the manuscript.

References

Bailey, G. B., and Presgrave, R. (1958). *Basic motion timestudy*. New York: McGraw-Hill.
Bainbridge, L., and Sanders, M. (1972). The generality of Fitts' Law. *Journal of Experimental Psychology, 96*, 130–133.
Begbie, G. H. (1959). Accuracy in timing in linear hand movements. *Quarterly Journal of Experimental Psychology, 21*, 65–75.
Beggs, W. D. A., and Howarth, C. I. (1970). Movement control in a repetitive motor task. *Nature, 225*, 752–753.
Beggs, W. D. A., and Howarth, C. I. (1972). The movement of the hand towards a target. *Quarterly Journal of Experimental Psychology, 24*, 448–453.
Beggs, W. D. A., and Howarth, C. I. (1972). The accuracy of aiming at a target: Some further evidence for a theory of intermittent control. *Acta Psychologica, 36*, 171–177.
Beggs, W. D. A., Graham, J. C., Monk, T. H., Shaw, M. R. W., and Howarth, C. I. (1972). Can Hick's Law and Fitts' Law be combined? *Acta Psychologica, 36*, 348–357.
Bergson, H. (1910). *Time and free will*. New York: Macmillan.
Brown, J. S., Knauft, E.B., and Rosenbaum, C. (1958). The accuracy of positioning reactions as a function of their direction and extent. *American Journal of Psychology, 61*, 167–182.
Carlton, L. G. (1979a). Control processes in the production of discrete aiming responses. *Journal of Human Movement Studies, 5*, 115–124.
Carlton, L. G. (1979b). *The role of vision for the control of aiming movements*. Unpublished Doctoral Dissertation, University of Illinois.
Carlton, L. G. (1980). Movement control characteristics of aiming responses. *Ergonomics, 23*, 1019–1032.
Carlton, L. G. (1981). Processing visual feedback information for movement control. *Journal of Experimental Psychology: Human Perception and Performance, 7*, 1019–1030.
Carlton, L. G., and Newell, K. M. (1985). *Response variability as a function of force parameters in dynamic tasks*. Manuscript in preparation.
Clausen, J. (1950). An evaluation of experimental methods of time judgment. *Journal of Experimental Psychology, 40*,756–761.
Craik, K. J. W., and Vince, M. A. (1963a). Psychological and physiological aspects of control mechanisms with special reference to tank gunnery I. *Ergonomics, 6*, 1–33.
Craik, K. J. W., and Vince, M. A. (1963b). Psychological and physiological aspects of control mechanisms II. *Ergonomics, 6*, 419–440.
Crossman, E. R. F. W., (1957). The speed and accuracy of simple hand movements. In E. R. F. W. Crossman and W. D. Seymour (Eds.), *The nature and acquisition of industrial skills*. Report to M. R. C. and D. S. I. R. Joint Committee on Individual Efficiency in Industry.
Crossman, E. R. F. W. and Goodeve, P. J. (1963). *Feedback control of hand movements and Fitts' Law*. Paper presented at the Experimental Psychology Meeting, Oxford, England, 1963. Published in *Quarterly Journal of Experimental Psychology 35A*, 251–278.
Drury, C. G. (1971). *Movements with lateral constraints*. Ergonomics,14, 239–305.
Ellis, M. J. (1969). Control dynamics and timing a discrete response. *Journal of Motor Behavior, 1*, 119–134.
Ellis, M. J., Schmidt, R. A., and Wade, M. G. (1968). Proprioception variables as determinants of lapsed-time estimation. *Ergonomics, 11*, 557–586.
Fitts, P. M. (1954). The information capacity of the human motor system in controlling the amplitude of movement. *Journal of Experimental Psychology, 47*, 381–391.
Fitts, P. M., and Peterson, J. R. (1964). Information capacity of discrete motor responses. *Journal of Experimental Psychology, 67*, 103–112.
Fullerton, G. S., and Cattell, J. McK. (1892). On the perception of small differences. *University of Pennsylvania Philosophical Series*, No. 2.
Garrett, H. E. (1922). A study of the relation of accuracy to speed. *Archives of Psychology, 8*, No. 56.

Hancock, W. M., Langolf, G., and Clark, D. O. (1973). Development of standard data for stereoscopic microscope work. *AIIE Transactions, 5*, 113–118.

Hoel, P. G. (1971). *Introduction to mathematical statistics* (4th ed.). New York: Wiley.

Howarth, C. I., Beggs, W. D. A., and Bowden, J. M. (1971). The relationship between the speed and accuracy of movement aimed at a target. *Acta Psychologica, 35*, 207–218.

Howells, R. A., Knight, J. L., Weiss, S. M., and Kak, A. V. (1979). Micro-timesharing within a single task. *Proceedings of the Human Factors Society Meeting, 23*, 523–526.

Jagacinski, R. J., Repperger, D. W., Ward, S. L., and Moran, M. S. (1980). A test of Fitts Law with moving targets. *Human Factors, 22*, 225–233.

Kantowitz, B. H., and Knight, J. L., Jr. (1978). Testing tapping time-sharing attention demands of movement amplitude target width. In G. E. Stelmach (Ed.), *Information processing in motor control and learning*. New York: Academic.

Keele, S. W. (1968). Movement control in skilled motor performance. *Psychological Bulletin, 70*, 387–403.

Keele, S. W., and Posner, M. I. (1968). Processing visual feedback in rapid movements. *Journal of Experimental Psychology, 77*, 155–158.

Kerr, B., and Langolf, G. D. (1977). Speed of aiming movements. *Quarterly Journal of Experimental Psychology, 19*, 474–481.

Kerr, R. (1973). Movement time in an underwater environment. *Journal of Motor Behavior, 5*, 175–178.

Klapp, S. T. (1975). Feedback versus motor programming in the control of aimed movements. *Journal of Experimental Psychology: Human Perception and Performance, 104*, 147–153.

Kvålseth, T. O. (1979). Note on information capacity of discrete motor responses. *Perceptual and Motor Skills, 49*, 291–296.

Kvålseth, T. O. (1980). An alternative to Fitts' Law. *Bulletin of the Psychonomic Society, 16*, 371–373.

Langolf, G. D., Chaffin, D. B., and Foulke, J. A. (1976). An investigation of Fitts' Law using a wide range of movement amplitudes. *Journal of Motor Behavior, 8*, 113–128.

Lee, D. N. (1980). Visuo-motor coordination in space-time. In G. E. Stelmach and J. Requin (Eds.), *Tutorials in motor behavior*. Amsterdam: North Holland.

Legge, D., and Barber, P. J. (1976). *Information and skill*. London: Methuen.

Locke, J. (1959). *An essay concerning human understanding*. Edited by A. C. Fraser. London: Dover. (Originally published 1690).

Meyer, D. E., Smith, J. E. K., and Wright, C. E. (1982). Models for the speed and accuracy of aimed limb movements. *Psychological Review, 89*, 449–482.

Michon, J. A. (1967). *Timing in temporal tracking*. Soesterberg, The Netherlands: Institute for Perception RVO-TNO.

Minkowski, H. (1923). Space and time, 1908. In H. A. Lorentz, A. Einstein, H. Minkowski, and H. Weyl (Eds.), *The principle of relativity*. London: Dover.

Newell, K. M. (1974). Knowledge of results and motor learning. *Journal of Motor Behavior, 6*, 235–243.

Newell, K. M. (1976). Motor learning without knowledge of results through the development of a response recognition mechanism. *Journal of Motor Behavior, 8*, 209–217.

Newell, K. M. (1980). The speed-accuracy paradox in movement control: Errors of time and space. In G. E. Stelmach and J. Requin (Eds.), *Tutorials in motor behavior*. Amsterdam: North Holland.

Newell, K. M., Carlton, L. G., Carlton, M. J. (1982). The relationship of impulse to timing error. *Journal of Motor Behavior, 14*, 24–45.

Newell, K. M., Carlton, L. G., and Hancock, P. A (1984). A kinetic analysis of response variability. *Psychological Bulletin, 96*, 133–151.

Newell, K. M., Carlton, M. J., Carlton, L. G., and Halbert, J. A. (1980). Velocity as a factor in movement timing accuracy. *Journal of Motor Behavior, 12*, 47–56.

Newell, K. M., and Hancock, P. A. (1984). Forgotten moments: Skewness and kurtosis as influential factors in inferences extrapolated from response distributions. *Journal of Motor Behavior, 16,* 320–335.

Newell, K. M., Hancock, P. A., and Robertson, R. N. (1984). A note on the speed-amplitude function in movement control. *Journal of Motor Behavior, 16,* 460–468.

Newell, K. M., Hoshizaki, L. E. F., Carlton, M. J., and Halbert, J. A. (1979). Movement time and velocity as determinants of movement timing accuracy. *Journal of Motor Behavior, 11,* 49–58.

Philip, B. R. (1936). The relationship between speed and accuracy in a motor task. *Journal of Experimental Psychology, 19,* 24–50.

Poulton, E. C. (1957). On prediction in skilled movement. *Psychological Bulletin, 54,* 467–478.

Schmidt, R. A. (1969). Movement time as a determiner of timing accuracy. *Journal of Experimental Psychology, 79,* 43–47.

Schmidt, R. A., and Russell, D. G. (1972). Movement velocity and movement time as determiners of the degree of preprogramming in simple movements. *Journal of Experimental Psychology, 96,* 315–320.

Schmidt, R. A., and Sherwood, D. E. (1982). An inverted-U relation between spatial error and force requirements in rapid limb movements: Further evidence for the impulse variability model. *Journal of Experimental Psychology: Human Perception and Performance, 8,* 158–170.

Schmidt, R. A., Zelaznik, H. N., and Frank, J. S. (1978). Sources of inaccuracy in rapid movement. In G. E. Stelmach (Ed.), *Information processing in motor control and learning.* New York: Academic.

Schmidt, R. A., Zelaznik, H. N., Hawkins, B., Frank, J. S., and Quinn, J. T. Jr. (1979). Motor output variability: A theory for the accuracy of rapid motor acts. *Psychological Review, 86,* 415–451.

Shannon, C. E., and Weaver, W. (1949). *The mathematical theory of communication.* Urbana: University of Illinois Press.

Sheridan, M. R. (1979). A reappraisal of Fitts' Law. *Journal of Motor Behavior, 11,* 179–188.

Sherwood, D. E., and Schmidt, R. A. (1980). The relationship between force and force variability in minimal and near-maximal static and dynamic contractions. *Journal of Motor Behavior, 12,* 75–89.

Siddall, G. J., Holding, D. H., and Draper, J. (1957). Errors of aim and extent in manual point to point movement. *Occupational Psychology, 31,* 185–195.

Smith, W. M., and Bowen, K. F. (1980). The effects of delayed and displaced visual feedback on motor control. *Journal of Motor Behavior, 12,* 91–102.

Tyldesley, D. A. (1980). The role of the movement structure in anticipatory timing. In G. E. Stelmach and J. Requin (Eds.), *Tutorials in motor behavior.* Amsterdam: North Holland.

Viviani, P., and Terzuolo, V. (1980). Space-time invariance in learned motor skills. In G. E. Stelmach and J. Requin (Eds.), *Tutorials in motor behavior.* Amsterdam: North Holland.

Wade, M. G., Newell, K. M., and Wallace, S. A. (1978). Decision time and movement time as a function of response complexity in retarded persons. *American Journal of Mental Deficiency, 63,* 135–144.

Wadman, W. J., Denier van der Gon, J. J., Geuze, R. H., and Mol, C. R. (1979). Control of fast goal directed arm movements. *Journal of Human Movement Studies, 5,* 3–17.

Wallace, S. A., Newell, K. M., and Wade, M. G. (1978). Decision and response times as a function of movement difficulty in preschool children. *Child Development, 49,* 509–512.

Weber, E. H. (1834). De pulsu, resorptione, auditu et tactu: Annotationes anatomicae et physiologicae. Leipzig: Koehler, 1834, R. J. Herrnstein and E. G. Boring (Eds.) *A source book in the history of psychology.* Cambridge, MA: Harvard University Press, 1965.

Welford, A. T. (1968). *Fundamentals of skill.* London: Methuen.
Welford, A. T., Norris, A. H., and Shock, N. W. (1969). Speed and accuracy of movement and their changes with age. In W. G. Koster (Ed.) *Attention and performance II.* Amsterdam: North Holland.
Wing, A. M., and Kristofferson, A. B. (1973a). The timing of interresponse intervals. *Perception and Psychophysics, 13,* 455–560.
Wing, A. M., and Kristofferson, A. B. (1973b). Response delays and the timing of discrete motor responses. *Perception and Psychophysics, 14,* 5–12.
Woodrow, H. (1951). Time perception. In S. S. Stevens (Ed.) *Handbook of experimental psychology.* New York: Wiley.
Woodworth, R. S. (1899). The accuracy of voluntary movements. *Psychological Review,* Monograph Supplement 3, Whole No. 13, No. 3.
Wright, C. E., and Meyer, D. E. (1983). Sources of the linear speed-accuracy trade-off in aimed movements. *Quarterly Journal of Experimental Psychology, 35A,* 279–296.

Motor Learning: A Review

JOHN ANNETT

Contents

Introduction

Motor learning is an expanding field and one in which theoretical perspectives are changing. This review will, therefore, be selective, making only passing reference to some of the classical topics such as feedback and transfer but focussing on what seem to me to be some of the important issues of the moment.

Practice makes perfect; yet there are techniques of instruction which can affect motor learning but which do not involve overt practice. These include demonstration and imitation, verbal instruction in rules and principles and imaginary or mental practice. In the first part of my paper I discuss these cognitive processes which can facilitate motor learning and describe some previously unpublished research. In the second part of the paper I discuss some current theories of practice, that is theories about the effects of repeatedly performing a task.

Cognitive Processes in Motor Learning

The distinction between cognitive and non-cognitive processes in motor learning was made by Fitts (1964). Although he cautiously spoke of a continuous process of skill learning he distinguished an "early" stage in which subjects learned what was required of them and an intermediate or associative phase which could involve the learning of cognitive sets. In the late phase of learning and especially with coherent tasks the skill becomes automatised and cognitive processes, such as verbal mediation, are no longer in evidence. Cognitive processes may be taken to be those which involve specific conscious experience and/or symbolic representation of crucial aspects of the task, but in the last analysis the only undeniable characteristic of cognitive processes is that they are covert. They have to do with overt actions and they may involve representations of overt actions but the actions themselves are inhibited.

Two kind of cognitive processes are of particular interest, those which involve analogue and those which involve symbolic representations. Thus the overt activity of say, jumping, may be cognitively represented by visual or kinaesthetic images of jumping and also by symbolic representations such as words like "jump", "hop", "leap" and so on. Both these kinds of representations can be present and can be manipulated covertly in various ways. That such manipulations can result in motor learning with measurable improvements in overt performance is not in question; what is my concern is the lack of any satisfactory theoretical account of these effects. I shall consider first recent evidence about the processes underlying mental practice and then the problem of how verbally coded information can impinge on motor learning.

Mental Practice

Much of the mental practice literature is unsatisfactory (see reviews by Corbin 1972, and Richardson 1967 a, b) but learning gains are reliably found and can sometimes be almost as great as those obtained by an equivalent amount of actual practice.

Two main types of theory have been advanced to account for mental practice effects. The first suggests that most real-life tasks include components of symbolic (verbalisable) and non-symbolic or perceptual-motor activity. The symbolically coded activity is capable of being rehearsed covertly and practice is able to strengthen these activities. The partial success of mental practice is therefore explained by this theory in terms of the relative importance of those aspects of the task which can be encoded symbolically. The second type of theory proposes that it is possible to inhibit motor activity at a very peripheral level. Mental practice then involves virtually all the neural activity associated with overt performance save some relatively trivial final motor output stage. Neither theory has a role for external feedback in learning and must therefore rely on hypothetical internal feedback or fall back, as Mackay (1981) proposes, on the law of exercise, as a sufficient principle for motor learning.

Mental practice is, by its very nature, difficult to control experimentally but a recent series of experiments by Johnson (1982) go some way towards overcoming this problem. There is a well-known effect in short-term memory for linear movement. A similar movement but of different extent interpolated between the learning trial and the recall trial will tend to introduce a constant error (CE) bias on recall. If the interpolated movement is shorter than the movement to be recalled then the latter is underestimated and if longer then the CE on recall will be one

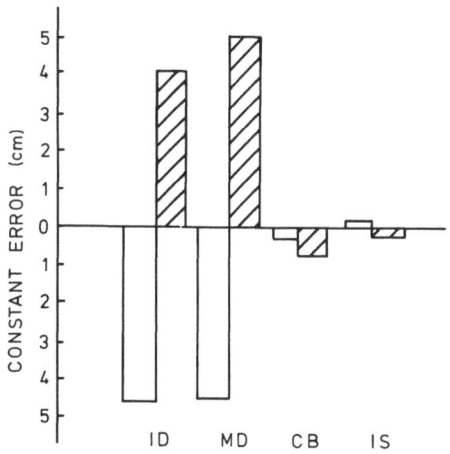

Fig. 1. Effects of interpolated activity on CE in motor STM. *ID*, imaginary movement different from standard; *MD*, real movement different from standard; *IS* imaginary movement same as standard; *CB*, counting backwards. The *hatched areas* represent the 30 cm standard and the plain 60 cm standard. (After Johnson 1982)

of overestimation. Johnson's subjects were required to learn either 30 or 60 cm by moving a slider 10 times along a rail to a stop set at one of these positions. They then did a further 10 trials under one of 4 conditions of interpolated practice. One of these conditions required subjects to make actual movements shorter or longer than the standard and in two others subjects were asked simply to imagine they were making a movement of the same extent, or only half as long or twice as long as the standard. A control group counted backwards in threes.

The results are shown in Fig. 1. The classic finding of over- and underestimation is clearly seen when the interpolated movement is shorter or longer than the original, with no bias on recall when the interpolated movement is of the same length. The striking feature of these results, however, is that the interpolated movement can be either real or imaginary but the effect is the same. In this experiment the imagined movement is, in the term used by Finke (1979), functionally equivalent to the real movement. It would appear that whatever memory trace is affected by the real movement is also affected by the imaginary movement.

The next step is to ask if this equivalence is total or if it can be analysed into components. The method used was to give the subjects a secondary task while attempting to follow instructions to execute the imaginary movements. We call this secondary interference since the primary effect is itself an interference effect. It is possible to infer something of the processes underlying the production of imaginary movements by the use of the secondary interference technique. For example, if the secondary task involves systems which directly control the relevant limb, requiring that limb to make a different movement would be expected to interfere with the imagery process. We can infer that the imagery has been affected not just by appealing to subjective evidence but by noting whether the imagery-induced bias is present or absent. A further experiment illustrates the method.

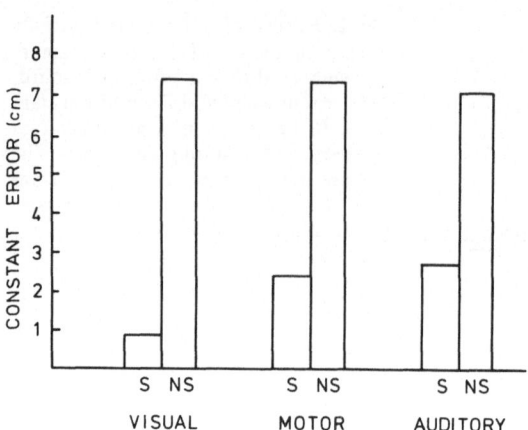

Fig. 2. Effect of secondary interference on CE in motor STM. *S,* spatial; *NS*, non-spatial

The task is basically the same as before except that subjects are required to carry out one of six secondary tasks whilst imagining the interpolated movement. Two of these tasks involved attending to visual stimuli, two involved attending to auditory stimuli and two required the subject to tap rhythmically with the hand involved in the imaginary movement either at one point or alternately at two widely separated points in the same plane as the imagined movement. The visual task required the subjects to watch a pair of lights flash on and off. In one case the lights were close together whilst in the other they were widely separated. The auditory tasks simply required the subjects to listen to a series of pulses generated by an electronic metronome, in one case from a single source in front of the subject and in the other coming alternately from loudspeakers placed to the right and left of the subject. Thus in each of these three pairs one task required the subject to attend to a single location whilst the other required attention to two spatially separated locations. The results are shown in Fig. 2.

A low value for CE indicates that the bias induced by the imaginary movement instructions has been eliminated and it can be seen that where the secondary task involves spatially separated events the bias is greatly reduced compared with those cases, regardless of modality, where only a single location is involved. In all three cases of "spatial" interference the CE bias is not significantly different from zero. The difference between the two motor tasks is instructive. It is possible to activate the limb used in imaginary practice without destroying the biasing effect of the imagery instructions and this result makes it extremely unlikely that the locus of the mental practice effect is in the peripheral motor system.

The systematic finding across all three modalities of secondary interference is that in tasks involving different spatial locations the imagery-induced bias is abolished so we may conclude that the imaginary movement involves a resource crucial to the representation of space which cannot be shared but does not involve resources required for the control of the musculature of that particular limb. We should nevertheless remember that the linear positioning task requires the representation of spatial locations and this may not be true of all tasks which can be mentally rehearsed.

In a very different context Mackay (1981) has demonstrated mental practice effects which also seem to preclude the influence of peripheral motor mechanisms. The skill in this case was reading sentences in English or German as fast as possible. The subjects were all bilingual and 12 sentences in each language were used. The times for reading these sentences were reduced with practice, including silent reading (which can be taken as mental practice). The particularly interesting result was that when subjects were required to read sentences which were either non-literal translations of the practice sentences (into German or English) or unrelated sentences there was significant transfer of training for the translations, but not for the unrelated sentences, and transfer was even greater for mental practice than for actual practice. Since reading the translated sentences involved totally different patterns of muscular activity an explanation in terms of peripheral innervation is ruled out.

Mackay advances a theory (described in greater detail in a later section) which proposes that sentence production involves a hierarchy of structures with those controlling the musculature at the lowest level and structures concerned with meaning and grammatical forms nearer the top of the hierarchy. Mackay suggests that during mental practice only the higher-level nodes are activated, but exercising these nodes has a strong effect since the higher they are the more uniquely they will be associated with any particular performance. For instance the systems controlling the lips and tongue are involved in all speech production and in other activities such as eating and are therefore well practised compared with structures concerned with expressing particular ideas or particular grammatical forms. Mackay's theory therefore attributes mental practice effects to a locus in the response organisation hierarchy well above that responsible for producing specific articulatory movements.

One of my students asked whether it was possible to narrow down the locus of MP effects in a motor task, a simple kind of tracking task which required the subject to follow an irregular zigzag track with a pencil. For this experiment the time for each trial was fixed at 10 s since unconstrained MP trials are often faster than actual trials, and so accuracy alone was scored as percentage time on the track. After pre-training on a standard track one group carried out 30 mental practice trials in which they were instructed to follow the same track, which remained visible, in their imagination and at the same constant speed, paced by an external timer. A second mental practice group had 30 trials in which they were asked to mentally follow 10 different tracks, each presented 3 times. A control group was given light reading material for an equivalent time between the initial training and the transfer task. Subjects were then tested on the original track. The no-practice control group failed to show significant improvement whilst each of the two other groups showed highly significant improvement. Although the group rehearsing on 10 different tracks showed marginally less improvement than those rehearsing on the single-test track the difference was not statistically significant.

The finding of this experiment, together with those of Johnson (1982) and Mackay (1981), are clearly incompatible with any theory which attributes mental practice effects to the activation of peripheral output mechanisms. Mental practice clearly involves the activation of some aspects of the internal representation of actions and in this task a representation which is more abstract than any specific pattern of overt hand or eye movements. What seems to be emerging is that the representations which are most effective in mental practice are of a rather abstract kind, such as spatial context in Johnson's experiments, core meaning in Mackay's experiments, and control rules rather than specific movements in the tracing experiment. If each of these rather different skills is thought of as being controlled by a motor plan then it would appear that rehearsal of critical and invariant elements of the plan which may be represented in imagery is the source of mental practice effects. The executive details of the plan, which may in any case have to be varied from time to time to meet variable conditions, probably contribute little and may not be laid down in a permanent store.

Action and Language

What Fitts (1964) called the "early phase" of skill learning includes understanding instructions. Instructors and coaches do at least part of their teaching by talking to their pupils and yet the process of translating between the verbal or symbolic code and the perceptual-motor or non-symbolic code has been largely unexplored (Annett 1983).

The relationship between the language system and the systems controlling action presents some problems of general significance to psychology and has been the subject of both speculation and experimental investigation (Kinsbourne 1981; Ornstein 1972). The popular "inner game" movement in sports coaching (Gallwey 1975) emphasises the distinction between verbal and non-verbal processes in a model of coaching characterised by a duality of the learner, who is said to comprise "Self 1", a verbal, logical, assertive individual concerned with the evaluation of achievement and "Self 2", who is non-verbal and intuitive and unconcerned about achievement. It is Self 2 which actually learns to perform skilful acts.

The "inner game" philosophy calls into question the value of verbal instruction and practice which is virtually devoid of tightly specified goals, and verbal evaluation is recommended. Simply hitting the ball, almost at random, allows Self 2 an uncluttered opportunity to acquire skilled perceptual-motor coordination. Inner game techniques have not been systematically evaluated but the following very informal experiment provides some insights into the nature of the relationship between the verbal and non-verbal domains in a motor skill. In Fig. 3 are some examples of verbal protocols collected while subjects were learning to perform a novel perceptual-motor task, either mirror tracing or pursuit rotor

"Left. Get the direction. Try not to wiggle too much. Ah, I've got the idea I think. I can't judge the distance too well. Now I've got to change my whole perspective. I want to come back on myself, I find. Thinks ... what have I got to do? Go the other way ... no I can't. I can't move. Right, what can I do?"

"Got to go backwards, so must go forwards. How many times does it take? I seem to stop and I can't move. Go back. If I go back I go forwards ... I seem to stop and I can't move ..."

"You can tell when it is absolutely catastrophic, which it was the last few times ... but you can tell when it was quite a good one as well ..."

"I do tend to consciously do it in an 'M' pattern now rather than a continuous line ...".

Fig. 3. Extracts from verbal protocols of subjects commenting simultaneously on mirror drawing and pursuit rotor performance

tracking. In some trials subjects were asked to say whatever came into their minds whilst performing the task.

The first observation of note is that whilst subjects feel that the dual task of talking and tracking requires some additional effort the two are not in serious competition. Neither level of performance nor rate of learning is affected by overt verbalisation about the task in hand as we might expect if we are indeed looking at two virtually independent systems. The content of the protocols does seem to bear out the duality of experience referred to by Gallwey. The "talking self" does not appear to be able to exert satisfactory control over the performing limb but nevertheless rapidly detects error and is generally critical, sometimes even downright annoyed, at the general level of achievement. There are occasional attempts to exert better control by imposing an abstractly formulated strategy on the recalcitrant limb, for example identifying the pattern of movement as an '*M*' in the pursuit rotor or explicitly stating the reversal rule in the mirror-drawing protocols.

There can be little doubt from inspecting these protocols that the verbal system is able to handle evaluation and make strategic suggestions but we do not know from these data whether the suggestions are actually beneficial or whether non-verbal learning progresses independently in its own way and at its own pace.

James (1890) proposed that verbal cognitive processes can play a significant role in the early learning of a skill but that highly practised performance is relatively inaccessible to influences from conscious verbal processes. Another small experiment bears on this question. Thirty-eight subjects who comprised four groups, non-swimmers, novices attending a beginner's class, casual swimmers and expert swimmers who were members of the University or County teams, were tested on their verbal knowledge of the breast stroke. Subjects were shown a series of cards carrying statements such as "as the arms push back the legs thrust backwards" and were required to respond "true" or "false" as quickly as possible. Each statement was offered twice, once in its "true" form and once in its "false" form and subjects were scored correct on that item only when they answered correctly to both forms. The results in Table 1 show that the novices answered more questions correctly than the experts although the only statistically significant pairwise comparison was at the 5% level between the novices and the casual swimmers.

Table 1. Test of verbal knowledge of breast stroke. Percentage correct answers and mean reaction times

	Non-swimmers	Casual swimmers	Novice class	Expert swimmers
Percentage correct	57.1	50.2	69.0	62.5
Response time (sec)	6.4	5.5	6.3	4.5

Reaction time to the questions was also measured by stopwatch and whilst the experts showed a faster mean reaction time (RT) than the non-swimmers ($p < 0.05$, one-tailed, on an a priori t-test) the groups did not differ significantly on a one-way analysis of variance. Subjects in all groups found this a rather difficult task and there is no clear evidence that degree of skill as such makes it more or less easy to translate between the verbal and the non-verbal domains. It could, of course, be argued that the cognitive content of a task such as swimming is in any case small but Adams (1981) has used a sequential switch-positioning task which was eminently capable of being verbalised or visualised and failed to find any evidence of reduced cognitive involvement after 200 trials of practice. His task was to set a row of twelve toggle switches in the "up" or "down" position according to an arbitrary pattern. Some subjects were given a similar verbal paired associate learning task of the form "1 up, 2 down . . . etc" just prior to learning the motor task whilst others were given the same interfering task after 200 learning trials. Adams found small and just significant interference effects on response times, but not on errors, both early and late in practice; thus both his experiment and mine fail to confirm the widely accepted story that skill acquisition is characterised by a progressive change in cognitive involvement.

Motor Imagery: A Bridge Between Action and Language

Given that there is a dissociation between verbal and perceptual-motor competencies translation between the two is nevertheless possible. Instructors can sometimes find expressions which convey relatively complex motor meanings. A colleague who coaches squash persuades his pupils to hold their rackets in readiness to receive service by telling them to "pretend to be a Red Indian on the warpath waving a tomahawk". This instruction, for most people in Britain, summons up a vividly remembered childhood image of the Hollywood caricature Indian and with it the required stance. It encapsulates what would otherwise be much longer statements specifying the angles of virtually all the main body joints as well as a feeling of tension and preparedness to act. At this level translation between the verbal symbolic code and the perceptual-motor code seems effortless and so it is worth enquiring how such a translation can take place when ordinarily the difficulty is considerable. Is there a special mediational mechanism or some kind of lingua franca which creates a functional bridge between action and language?

The converse of following instructions is to give explanations or directions and so one kind of investigation which may shed light on the nature of verbal-motor communication is to ask subjects to provide explanations of how to carry out actions with which they are familiar. In a series of experiments, which are still in progress, subjects were given instructions such as "tell me in as much detail as you can how you mount and ride away on a bicycle", "take two ends of string and tie them together to make a bow", and "perform a forward roll".

Two things are immediately apparent in subjects' responses to such requests. First they either close their eyes or look away from the experimenter's face. These are the immediate behavioural signs of imaging. Second, subjects make tentative movements as in grasping handlebars or pieces of string. Despite this compulsion to gesture it would appear that overt movement is not in fact critical to the production of explanation, but when overt performance is inhibited imagery is absolutely essential to the production of a verbal explanation.

In different experimental conditions I have employed secondary tasks which might be expected to interfere with some aspects of the process or special conditions which might be expected to facilitate the generation of an explanation as measured by simple indices such as its length, duration and accuracy. For example, subjects required to tap on the table top with the preferred hand at a rate of once per second showed very little difference from control subjects in any of the three indices, including accuracy of the explanation. Imagery is not mentioned in the instructions, nor in the invitation to subjects to participate in the experiments. After completing their descriptions subjects answered a detailed questionnaire on the imagery they experienced and from their replies some interesting characteristics have emerged. Most subjects report imagery which is predominantly visual rather than tactile or kinaesthetic.

This paucity of tactile and kinaesthetic imagery is rather surprising in view of the nature of the tasks. For example when giving a description of bow-tying subjects readily report the colour of the string but cannot say whether it felt rough or smooth nor any feelings of tension associated with pulling the string tight. When asked to describe a forward roll some subjects report a feeling of pressure on the neck and back. The reported visual imagery is usually quite specific where concerned with essentials but vague in other respects. Some subjects, for instance, image the laces of a particular pair of shoes and when describing the forward roll frequently report on the surface on which the feat is performed, often a particular rug or carpet at home or a gymnasium mat or perhaps the lawn in their own garden. The clothing worn by the performer is often described in detail although it is not essential to the description and never features in it.

Another feature of the imagery is that it is normally egocentric, that is visualised as if through one's own eyes, but sometimes individuals visualise themselves performing the task from an external viewpoint, as if on a video recorder. This is reported most commonly in describing the forward roll where sometimes the imagery can switch back and forth between the egocentric and outside viewpoints during the course of a description. The imagery is to some extent controllable in the sense that subjects report being able to slow it down or speed it up but going into reverse or envisaging stages separately in other than the normal order is rarely attempted and appears to be difficult; indeed one of the main problems for subjects is to keep their place. Occasionally the image is lost, not always as the result of an external distractor, and subjects then have to recreate the image, sometimes going back to the beginning of the operation, before being able to continue with their description. Performance on this type of task is fairly resistant to simple motor, visual, and auditory distractors but is also not much affected by conditions one might think would be helpful. For instance in one condition subjects were given 30 s warning of the description they were to produce. Another group was given a piece of wood with two pieces of string attached and asked to make a bow. This was then removed and subjects were required to give their description. Finally one group was given the board with the string and asked to give their description whilst actually tying the bow. No significant difference was found between any of these conditions and the standard condition in the number of words used, the time taken or the accuracy of the descriptions. In fact the transcriptions of subjects' descriptions are indistinguishable except for differences in tense. Subjects relying on imagery normally say "I would" or "you should" whilst those relying on recent memory tend to use the past tense, describing what they have just done and those actually performing the task use the present, or occasionally the future, tense.

Discussion

The most important issue raised by these studies is that of the form of representation of motor competence. It is possible to construct in broad outline a theoretical account of the significant relationships between perceptual, motor, verbal and imaginal processes which may be active in skill acquisition. The protocols from the "talk as you track" situation and the descriptions experiments illustrate the dissociation between the verbal and motor codes even to the point at which Gallwey's description of Self 1 and Self 2 does not seem entirely fanciful.

How then does verbal instruction influence skill acquisition? It is possible to conceive, at least in principle, a common or neutral code, perhaps something like Pylyshyn's (1981) propositional form in which motor memories, or the capabilities for performing tasks, may be stored. If these are stored in a sufficiently general form the capacity for tying bows might be adaptable to a wider range of specific outputs, say using different kinds of string and rope in varied circumstances and, if really general, might be capable of being translated into a verbal code just as information stored in a computer can be output in digital or analogue form or used to control a number of different output devices. This analogy does not seem to fit the storage of motor performance capability. The systems capable of producing language output need to monitor the output, real or imagined, of other systems which possess motor competences in order to be able to translate from the motor to the verbal code; they might almost be observing the actions of another individual. The ability to translate in the opposite direction, from verbal to motor, is not very powerful as is shown by the comments of subjects who try to control their own mirror drawing or tracking behaviour. The exception seems to be when particularly vivid images are evoked, such as the Indian with the tomahawk. It seems that there are some action concepts which are readily accessible to the verbal system in this way but they may require the mediation of images.

By contrast the relationship between action and action imagery appears to be particularly intimate such that imaging an action can have effects on the memory trace equivalent to those of an overt action as was shown by Johnson's experiments. The very efficacy of coaching tricks of the "Red Indian with a tomahawk" type may depend on the intimacy of this relation between actions and their representations. If an appropriate form of words can summon an image then the image also seems to have power to summon the action. We see the counterpart of this process in the experiment where the internal rehearsal of actions generates images which can then be described and translated into a verbal code.

Actions, whether they be simple linear movements or more complex like tying a knot, seem to benefit from a kind of dual coding in which some aspects are capable of being represented in images, principally visual in nature and which represent important spatial characteristics of the task. At the same time there may be a "pure" motor code which is not accessible to consciousness but is only manifest in the ability to produce actions. Under normal circumstances actions are produced, probably with frequent monitoring, and verification of outcomes and what enters consciousness is the perceptual representations of these checks. When required to give descriptions of actions with motor output suppressed, perceptual traces of former actions are represented in imagery and it is these which the subject is able to describe. These functional relationships merit further investigation perhaps on the lines suggested by Annett (1983). For example, if the action-language bridge is a two-way system, difficulties in following instructions should be found to be matched by difficulties in giving instructions. Studies are needed of how action statements are understood and interpreted and what features of actions are describable.

Some Current Theories of Practice

Much of what we know about motor performance is derived from studies of the early stages of practice in which subjects practise unfamiliar tasks for at most a few hours. In the real world after months or years of practice typists and concert pianists produce performances which, if found under laboratory conditions, could be interpreted as evidence of enormously expanded information-processing capacity. In a wide variety of tasks in which time to complete a unit of behaviour is the dependent variable the logarithm of performance time decreases as a linear function of the logarithm of the number of practice trials. This relationship was pointed out by Crossman (1959) and the evidence has recently been reviewed by Mazur and Hastie (1978) and by Newell and Rosenbloom (1981). We now consider some of the hypotheses advanced to account for this relationship.

First we shall consider a modern variation on the classic notion of "engraining", that is the facilitation of behavioural, and presumably neural, pathways by sheer use. MacKay's (1982) theory is the most recent version of the old "law of exercise". Next there is a tradition of theories derived from the observations of Bryan and Harter (1899), which depends on the principle of "grouping", that is the absorption of small segments of behaviour into macro-units which can be dealt with as efficiently as their individual components but contain more information. The modern version of this theory has been espoused by Newell and Rosenbloom (1981) under the principle of "chunking". This theory may be distinguished from the hypothesis that practice is characterised by a progressive change in the level of control from "closed loop" to "open loop" as suggested by Poulton (1957) and developed by Pew (1966, 1974) and by Schneider, Shiffrin and others (Schneider and Fisk 1982).

A New Law of Exercise

Mackay's theory was developed in the context of speech production, including reading, and seeks to explain fluency and flexibility in serial skills. It includes specific proposals for a learning mechanism which gives an account of both overt and mental practice effects. Performance is mediated by a structure which is hierarchically organised in the manner shown in Fig. 4.

When a sentence is produced the structure is activated from the top down, the activity spreading downwards through the connected nodes represented by the boxes. At the top of the hierarchy there are nodes representing propositions, concepts, and lexical rules. As an intermediate level there is a hierarchy of structures from syllables to phonological features which are in turn connected to the relevant muscle movements required to produce a particular sequence of sounds.

At the conceptual level the basic proposition can be decomposed into noun phrase and verb phrase and at the phonological level syllables unpack into the initial consonant and vowel group and so on. At each of these three levels the set of nodes is governed by a timing mechanism and a network of syntactic rules. Thus at the conceptual level we have a system which assembles grammatical elements in the correct order and timing and so converts the basic proposition into a statement. The statement is not necessarily uttered aloud but may be subvocal

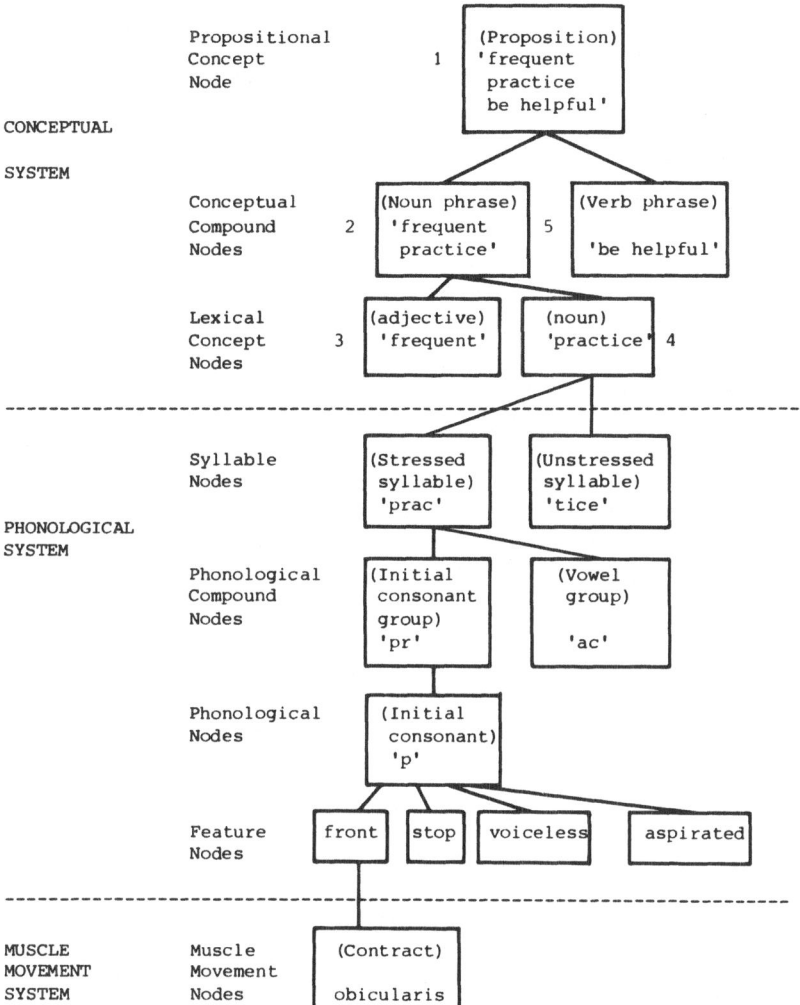

Fig. 4. The hierarchy of speech control systems. (After Mackay 1982)

or simply "thought" if the muscle activation system at the bottom of the hierarchy is not activated.

In overt behaviour the activation spreads downwards but in a way which is controlled at each level by the rules of ordering and timing; thus nodes 3 and 4 must be activated before node 5 and so on down through the system. A notable feature of the theory is that at the top of the hierarchy where sentences are constructed to express ideas there is generally rather little repetition whilst lower down the hierarchy where individual words are produced there may be a great deal of repetition, since common words are used many thousands of times during the course of a lifetime.

The basic assumption of the theory is that whenever a node is activated in the course of producing a sentence, whether it be a high-level conceptual node or a low-level phonological node, it primes all the other nodes to which it is connected. Priming may fall short of full activation but its effect is to speed up production so that when the lexical concept node "practice" is activated the stressed and the unstressed syllable nodes are primed but the unstressed syllable, controlled by the rules of ordering and timing, is not activated until both the initial consonant and the vowel (pr-ac) have been activated. This feature reflects the tendency for phonological elements to be run off more quickly when they occur near the end of a long word than at the beginning.

The theory gives a plausible account of a number of empirical phenomena (Mackay 1982), including the log-log linear improvement in the maximum rate at which words can be uttered. Learning is fast initially because the relatively unpractised high-level nodes contribute most to improvement. This follows from the presumed exponential growth of node priming with repetition. Normal sentences can be produced faster than scrambled sentences due to a well-established node structure at the conceptual level.

The theory also predicts the qualitative pattern of speed-error trade-off typical of skills in which speed is emphasised. A node is triggered when its priming summates and exceeds that of all the others in that domain. Given the assumption that activation is noisy the wrong node is sometimes triggered but the errors are far from random. The majority of substitutions are from the same category, noun for noun and verb for verb, and errors at the conceptual level tend also to be conceptually related. Because the strength of extraneous nodes which may cause the wrong node to be triggered decreases over time, whereas the correct or intended node increases in strength, delay will reduce the chance of error and in this way speed trade-off against error.

The theory also suggests an explanation of some mental practice and transfer of training phenomena. In mental practice the muscle nodes are inhibited but higher-level nodes can be activated and the "law of exercise" can operate to change the rate of priming of these nodes. Similarly in transfer (between hands, for example) high-level nodes will be activated even though quite different sets of effector muscles may be employed. Skills which are conceptually complex but with well-practised motor components should therefore show greater benefits from mental practice than those which involve unfamiliar movements but are relatively simple at the conceptual level and transfer should be greater between tasks which have common elements at a higher level in the underlying structure.

The problem in testing such a theory is to operationalise the concepts of "complexity" and "level". Mackay's theory is fundamentally connectionist but is more sophisticated than classical stimulus-response theories in that it allows for flexibility rather than rigidity to emerge from repeated practice.

An account of flexibility is a clear requirement for any comprehensive theory of motor learning as Schmidt (1975) pointed out in proposing his schema theory. The two theories, however, achieve flexibility in fundamentally different ways. In Schmidt's theory the schema is an abstraction of the relationships between arrays of information about a series of similar but not identical responses which permits the generation of further responses of the same type such as tennis shots. In Mackay's theory behaviour is generated by a hierarchy of systems, conceptual, phonological and muscular each of which is independently capable of benefiting from practice and being combined in many different ways to produce new response patterns.

Response Selection and Chunking

Crossman's theory of the acquisition of speed skills was based on the principle of selection of responses on the basis of the amount of time and/or effort they require. It is well known (see Rabbitt 1981) that the main effect of practice on speeded responses is to change the shape of their distribution. There is normally little change with practice in the fastest time recorded but the tail of long response latencies (or interresponse intervals) is reduced.

Mazur and Hastie (1978) have argued that if the mechanism underlying this change is the replacement of unsatisfactory responses by more efficient responses then the learning curve should be exponential but if correct, or more satisfactory, response tendencies increase and simply compete with incorrect response tendencies then the learning curve should be hyperbolic. The choice between these two variants of the selection theory may, in principle, be determined empirically. However, both versions give tolerably good predictions but the experimental data themselves often present problems by the absence of good estimates of origin and asymptote. There is also the question of whether individual learning curves resemble the group data to which the equations have typically been applied.

Whilst some impressively close fits have been reported by Newell and Rosenbloom (1981), a truly satisfactory theory would have to account for not just the fit of the learning curve but also the changes in response time distributions as demonstrated, for example, by Long, Nimmo-Smith and Whitfield (1983). Unfortunately few investigators report their data in sufficient detail to permit measures of changes in the second and third moments about the mean.

Newell and Rosenbloom having considered the closeness of fit of the range of functions conclude that the data from a number of sources do fit the family of generalised power functions and propose that the underlying mechanism which applies to all forms of learning task in which completion time is at a premium is that of "chunking". "Chunks" are structural units in the environment; thus a pattern of dots and dashes in morse code might be a chunk viewed either as input or output. The important feature of chunking is that primitive chunks can be combined into higher-order chunks which can be processed as "wholes" with a resultant saving in processing time. Newell and Rosenbloom propose that the chunking process generates a power law which closely fits the data in a variety of tasks ranging from problem solving and the perception of chessboard positions to perceptual-motor skills.

We may ask if chunking is purely a theoretical construct or whether it is possible to observe directly chunking processes in real tasks. To do this a fine-grained analysis is required and some studies of the acquisition of typewriting by Rumelhart and Norman (1982) provide suitable examples.

A skilled typist working at 200 words/minute may produce interresponse intervals of as little as 60 ms which are clearly far too short to allow for the serial processes of the classical linear information-processing model. Such speed can only be achieved if perception and response preparation can overlap with execution. One way in which speed is increased is by one hand beginning to move towards a target key before the other hand has completed its stroke and this can be seen on film records. Novices type repeat digraphs such as *oo* or *ee* faster than other digraphs whilst for the skilled typist inter-keystroke intervals tend to be more uniform. Rumelhart and Norman suggest the novice only conceptualises the double letters as units, each letter representing an individual location problem for the novice which in the case of double letters only has to be solved once. The more skilled the typist the greater the range of digraphs processed as pairs and the more it would seem that performance is limited by motor rather than cognitive constraints.

Examination of differences in error patterns between novices and well-practised performers by Grudin (1983) revealed something of the different ways in which the skill is organised. In novices, striking the wrong key which is the mirror image of the correct key, but in the wrong hand, was found to be relatively common (62% of errors) but this is much reduced (17%) with extensive practice. Transposition errors such as *hte* for *the* also change with practice. In novices most transposition errors occur within hands whilst in experts most transposition errors occur between hands.

Many of these features of the development of skill may be understood in terms of a model presented by Rumelhart and Norman (1982) based on a system of activated trigger schemas. Schemas, conceived essentially as flexible motor programs, are formed by experience and are triggered by their appropriate stimuli. The population of schemas are in contention with one another for execution. For example in typing the word *very* the movement to *v* from a standard position is down and to the right but this is in conflict with the next letter *e*, which requires a movement up and towards the left by the same hand, and so if the correct order is to be maintained the activation of *v* must inhibit *e*. The competition between *r* and *y* is minimal because different hands are used.

Rumelhart and Norman have devised a computer simulation which models the contention scheduling of these schemas. The model drives a pair of simulated hands across a keyboard by computing the moment-to-moment discrepancy between target position and actual finger position and using this information in conjunction with the activation levels of the individual keypress schemas to trigger responses. The process of activation and target discrepancy computation is recursive and continues until the target schema is within tolerance and the key is then struck.

The simulation is found to produce some of the characteristic features of skilled typing. For example short inter-keystroke intervals are achieved and, as with real typists, they are shorter between than within hands, basically because successive keystrokes within the same hand tend to pull it away from the next target key. Transposition errors occur mostly across hands for the same basic reason, that the next finger on the alternate hand has a speed advantage and is therefore more likely to be activated prematurely.

The Rumelhart and Norman simulation does not itself learn but rather simulates the already skilled typist. Perhaps its most interesting feature is that it accounts for the speed of skilled typing in terms of a fairly low-level mechanism whereby control of the keypressing movements is carried out relatively locally and in parallel.

The model seems to imply the operation of at least two distinguishable learning processes and it is arguable whether both constitute instances of "chunking". Grudin (1983) refers to the process by which the skilled typist, but not the novice, treats digrams other than doubles as groups as evidence of a cognitive component in learning, clearly an instance of chunking. The second process which gives rise to overlap of perceptual and response processes is conceptualised as a shift from central to more peripheral control where parallel processing is possible. The process of contention scheduling as between two activated letter schemas may also be thought of as a kind of chunking since the processes within any "chunk" are by definition autonomous. If so the model can be interpreted as implying two kinds of chunking which contribute to learning by two distinct processes, the grouping of inputs into global units and the delegation of motor control to lower centres.

Changes in Control Level

The delegation principle was envisaged by Poulton (1957) and has been elaborated by Pew (1966, 1974). For example, in tracking a regular sine wave the control problem is simplified if the three principal parameters of frequency, amplitude and phase are monitored and controlled in turn rather than attempting to respond to each deviation of the target on a moment-to-moment basis. Pew describes this process as attending to different higher-order variables and outputting motor control commands more as parameter adjustments than as detailed motor programmes.

Shaffer's (1981) account of skilled piano playing, like Grudin's description of the development of typing, requires two levels of representation, a cognitive representation of the input (or "input string") and a representation of the motor output or ("command string"). Shaffer demonstrated that skilled pianists can play a piece in strict time or with rubato and variations in emphasis to convey mood and feeling. These high-level features of the performance are represented in the input string as conscious intentions which can be influenced by both cognitive and emotional factors. This level of representation can be variable, and even creative, as in the case of improvisation. The command string, however, is slaved to the input string such that the input once formulated is executed automatically by the cerebellar-spinal system. This dual representation thus offers two kinds of opportunities for learning, one in the perception or appreciation of the intention and another in tuning up the output system such that its calculations are performed more efficiently. Shaffer conjectures that the role of kinaesthesis is to control and maintain the precision of the computational procedures which comprise in the output string.

Evidence for this kind of interpretation is derived from analysing detailed computer recordings of the timing of keystrokes during performances and in particular looking at the control of musical expression by systematic variations in the timing and rhythmic features of the performance (Shaffer 1981). For example, one professional pianist showed variations of as much as 2 to 1 in the duration of musical bars within a piece. This was not error since the same variations were found in a repeat performance. Furthermore this ability to reproduce complex temporal patterns could not have been due to the operation of a fixed motor program since the same pianist on a different occasion produced a significantly different, but equally valid, interpretation of the piece. The command string is nevertheless the slave of the input string, as shown by another performer who produced a fluent, correctly timed and accurate performance of an unseen piece after a quick glance through the score.

Automatic and Controlled Processing

In the typing and piano-playing examples a high degree of skill is characterised by performances which appear to be both autonomous and flexible. This is a critical point for motor learning theories since one view of the automatisation which comes with practice is that "open-loop" operation necessarily entails inflexibility. The series of studies by Schneider and Shiffrin (see Schneider and Fisk 1982; Shiffrin and Dumais, 1981) emphasise the dependence of automatisation on regularity of practice materials. For example, in a task in which subjects search visual displays for specified target items it is found that search time is a function of the size of the memory set only when the memory set is changed from trial to trial. After extended practice with an unchanged memory set search time becomes progressively faster and independent of set size.

Schneider and Shiffrin propose that there are two modes of processing, controlled and automatic. Performance on many tasks may involve both types but practice enables more processes to become automatic provided conditions are right, particularly if stimuli are consistently mapped onto responses. Automatic processing is characterised as fast, parallel, fairly effortless, unlimited by short-term memory capacity and not under voluntary control. Controlled processing, on the other hand, is slow, serial and limited by short-term memory capacity.

Much of the experimental work has been carried out on visual search tasks where the response is to identify one or more target letters in a display, but automatic processing has also been demonstrated in a serial motor task (Schneider and Eberts 1980). Eight buttons were pressed according to a sequence of eight digits and practice was either consistent with the same sequence on each trial or inconsistent, with one of several different sequences in random order on each trial. Subjects were required to tap a key simultaneously at a rate of 2/s. The accuracy of button pressing in the consistent sequence improved steadily whilst that in the inconsistent sequence did not. Interresponse intervals remained variable for the inconsistent sequences but variability was greatly reduced with the regular sequences. This empirical result is hardly surprising since learning one list of about the normal short-term memory capacity must be easier than seven such lists, even if each individual list received the same number of practice trials.

A consequence of automatisation is, presumably, the release of processing resources to cope with secondary tasks. The button-pressing task just described could be performed concurrently with a visual category search task after extensive practice provided the latter involved consistent mapping. Such a result is consistent with the demonstration of Allport et al. (1972) of dual-task performance in skilled pianists and also with Hirst et al. (1980) on simultaneous reading and taking dictation. The interpretation of these results is hotly debated. The Shiffrin and Schneider interpretation of "automatisation" may be contrasted with Neisser's view that improved performance with practice is accounted for as a real increase in capacity (Neisser, Hirst and Spelke 1981). The difference between these two positions may not be as great as first appears but hinges on the interpretation of what it means to pay conscious attention to performing a task. Schneider and Shiffrin's concept of automatisation, like that of Norman and Shallice (1980), defines automatic processes as "unconscious" or without awareness. For example, most people can walk over even ground whilst conducting a conversation or solving mental problems. A test of whether a process is automatic can then be carried out by assessing how much information has been processed in sufficient depth to have entered long-term memory. Hirst et al. (1980) were indeed able to demonstrate that there was a reasonable degree of comprehension of their dual-task material, reinforcing the view that some, if not all, the material had entered consciousness and had been processed enough to have been registered in long-term memory.

Shiffrin's suggestion that the result simply shows that comprehension itself can become automatised is unsatisfactory since it broadens the definition of automatisation to the point at which it is no longer distinguishable from controlled processing. The distinction between the two types of processing, at first sight attractive, does not permit clear differential predictions where they are most needed.

Discussion

The near universality of the log-log linear law of learning suggests that it must derive from some rather basic learning process such as "chunking" which can be understood in psychological or even neurological terms. But the simplicity of the log-log linear law is not necessarily the result of a single fundamental process. Similar "learning" curves typically occur in complex systems containing many elements which can change and in which there is a premium on time or effort. Such systems may or may not be organisms capable of learning in the psychological sense.

For instance, learning curves can be found in the development of new industrial production systems where the elements include people, machines, administrative procedures and a variety of different resources and processes each of which is capable of some degree of change, including substitution. A single dependent variable such as weekly output is governed by a variety of factors including familiarity of the operators with the equipment, reduction in down time as new equipment is debugged, improvements in the supply of materials and components, refinement of administrative procedures and many others which combine in small or large measure to improve performance.

The creation of records in sport provides another example of apparent learning in a complex system. New records are set when new solutions are found to any of many problems such as physiological fitness, training regime, technique, or equipment. The rate of improvement can be expected to slow down as a function of the number of ways there are left to improve and how much effort is put into their discovery. An individual practising a skill under time pressure is just another complex system exploiting possible ways of improving.

The detailed studies of typewriting referred to earlier show evidence of different kinds of performance changes as might be expected on this view. The progressive change in the timing patterns of diagraphs reported by Grudin appear to be an example of "chunking" but other changes contribute to the overall increase in speed. Long et al. (1983) deduce from detailed analyses of the shape of interresponse interval distributions that not only do fast responses get faster as the distributions become more peaked but the tail of slow responses is also reduced, apparently because visual checks on keyboard locations with which they are associated are progressively reduced in number. The eyes, as a limited information-processing resource, can spend more time dealing with the input text if less time is required recalibrating the spatial plan of the keyboard, which must serve as an input to the individual finger and hand movements.

It may be objected that it is unparsimonious to attribute the log-log linear law to an indefinitely large number of different sources of improvement with practice as opposed to a single mechanism such as Newell's chunking or Mackay's priming. This objection has some force if all the information we have is a plot of mean response times against practice trials, but more detailed analyses of the kind demonstrated by Grudin and Long et al. are capable of revealing the operation of different mechanisms. The widely accepted view that a principal source of improvement in performance is due to a progressive change from closed-loop to open-loop operation, or from controlled to automatic processing, has been questioned by Neisser et al. (1981) on the grounds that the increased capacity to execute two tasks simultaneously can be shown to be achieved without either rapid time sharing or by performing one task automatically.

The experiments by Adams (1981) which demonstrated that interference from cognitive processes did not vary as a function of practice tend to add further doubts about the classical story as does my experiment, described in the first section of this review, which showed skilled and novice swimmers about equally bad at describing in detail what their arms and legs were doing. Far from performance becoming more automatic, or less subject to voluntary control, as skill develops it often appears that practice enables the learner to bring involuntary actions under voluntary control. This can be seen clearly in mirror drawing when early in practice subjects experience considerable frustration when their hands refuse to move in the desired direction. In many sports and the performing arts a high degree of skill is characterised by an increasingly high degree of voluntary control over bodily movements. The development of sensorimotor coordination in children is similarly the progressive attainment of voluntary control over initially involuntary movements.

This paradox has its origins in the confusion which still surrounds the concept of attention. Allport (1980) in his cogent review of the issues suggests that the concept of a central channel of limited capacity has been misleading. Particular patterns of inter-task interference may be interpreted as evidence for the existence of specialised subsystems. If, as argued above, improvement with practice is essentially the result of the modification of contributary subsystems then the selection of strategies involving subsystems which do not interfere with a second task will sometimes, but not always, be possible. It is interesting to note that in the Hirst, Spelke and Neisser experiments the two competing tasks were already highly practised and there is no suggestion that extended practice improved performance in either significantly. The improvement was in their joint performance. There is absolutely no need to suppose that practice made either task less demanding of the available pool of that special commodity we call "attention".

But there is another important aspect to the problem of attention and control. There is a simple sense in which a skilled typist can be said to be "paying attention" to the text to be transcribed rather than to the positioning of the fingers on the keyboard. In the Rumelhart and Norman simulation finger location is determined by "local" computation. In terms of the standard story, assimilation of the text is a function of the limited channel whilst the moment-to-moment movements of the hands are determined by automatic processes which do not demand attention. Long et al. suggest that the skilled typist has an internal reference plan of the keyboard which is sufficiently reliable not to require frequent and time-consuming location checks. Whether the location problem is solved by reference to external visual space or to an internal plan the computation could equally be "automatic". It would be misleading to argue that hunt-and-peck typing is "controlled" whilst touch typing is "automatic" or that the process of learning is the automatisation of a previously conscious process when all that has happened is that a process which carries a time penalty (an extra visual fixation) has been eliminated.

Summary

In this rather selective review of motor learning I have chosen to dwell on a limited number of issues, distinguishing broadly between early learning and factors which mediate learning almost independently of overt practice, and later learning which is much more dependent on the sheer amount of practice and repetition. Understanding the mechanisms of mental practice could lead to a better understanding of the coding of movement information in the nervous system. Evidence is accumulating that the internal manipulation of relatively abstract imaginal representations of tasks can sometimes produce effects as powerful as those achieved by overt practice. The nature of these representations may vary from task to task but their locus appears to be closer to those centres which originate movement plans than to the peripheral executive mechanisms.

Imagery also appears to play an important role in mediating between the verbal-symbolic system and the motor system. Effective verbal instructions are those which evoke clear images whilst, conversely, the ability to perform a motor task can only be translated into the verbal code via the medium of imagery which is largely visual.

Recent evidence casts doubt on the long-held belief that motor skills are initially subject to conscious, cognitive, even verbal, control and that this kind of control diminishes progressively as a function of extended practice to give way to automatic processes. The verbal and motor systems are largely independent and the degree of their independence does not appear to be much affected by practice. However, the relations between overt motor activity and the imaginal and verbal-symbolic representation of action merit more research.

At the other end of the motor-learning continuum the effects of large amounts of practice have recently received renewed attention. The empirical log-log linear law of practice challenges interpretation. Candidates for a single underlying process include a new version of the law of exercise, the combination of units of behaviour into progressively larger "chunks" and the delegation of conscious cognitive control to automatic processes which make no demand on central processing capacity. Although automatisation can occur it is far from certain that it can account for all highly skilled performance since there is evidence that conscious control may be increased rather than decreased with practice.

Some of the recent studies of highly developed keyboard skills suggest a more complex picture in which several different processes contribute to the reduction of unit time for a given performance level, sometimes at the cost of particular error patterns. A conservative working hypothesis is that the log-log linear law is a general feature of complex systems in which constituent subsystems can be modified in response to environmental demands for efficiency. The alternative that the log-log linear law depends on the operation of a single psychological mechanism is clearly not yet proven.

Acknowledgement. Some of the work reported in this paper was supported by grants from the Social Science Research Council.

References

Adams, J. A. (1981). Do cognitive factors in motor performance become non-functional with practice? *Journal of Motor Behaviour, 13*, 262–273.

Allport, D. A. (1980). Attention and performance. In G. Claxton (Ed.) *Cognitive psychology: New directions.* London: Routledge and Kegan Paul.

Allport, D. A., Antonis, B., and Reynolds, P. (1972). On the division of attention: a disproof of the single channel hypothesis. *Quarterly Journal of Experimental Psychology, 24*, 225–235.

Annett, J. (1983). Motor learning: a cognitive psychological viewpoint. In H. Rieder, K. Bos, H. Mechling, and K. Reischle (eds.) *Motor learning and movement behavior. A contribution to learning in sport.* Schorndorf: Verlag Karl Hofmann.

Bryan, W. L., and Harter, N. (1899). Studies on the telegraphic language. The acquisition of a hierarchy of habits. *Psychological Review, 6*, 345–375.

Corbin, C. B. (1972). Mental practice. In W. D. Morgan (Ed.) *Ergogenic aid and muscular performance.* New York: Academic.

Crossman, E. R. F. W. (1959). A theory of the acquisition of speed-skill. *Ergonomics, 2*, 153–166.

Finke, R. A. (1979). The functional equivalence of mental images and errors of movement. *Cognitive Psychology, 11*, 235–264.

Fitts, P. M. (1964). Perceptual motor skill learning. In A. W. Melton (Ed.) *Categories of human learning.* New York: Academic.

Gallwey, W. T. (1975). *The inner game of tennis.* London: Cape.

Grudin, J. T. (1983). Error patterns in skilled and novice transcription typing. In W. E. Cooper (Ed.) *Cognitive aspects of skilled typewriting.* New York: Springer.

Hirst, W., Spelke, E. S., Reaves, C. C., Canarack, G., and Neisser, U. (1980). Dividing attention without alteration or automaticity. *Journal of Experimental Psychology: General, 109*, 98–117.

James, W. (1890). *The principles of psychology.* New York: Holt.

Johnson, P. (1982). The functional equivalence of imagery and movement. *Quarterly Journal of Experimental Psychology, 34 A*, 349–365.

Kinsbourne, M. (1981). Single channel theory. In D. Holding (Ed.) *Human skills.* Chichester: Wiley.

Long, J., Nimmo-Smith, I., and Whitefield, A. (1983). Skilled typing: a characterisation based on the distribution of times between responses. In W. E. Cooper (Ed.) *Cognitive aspects of skilled typewriting.* New York: Springer.

Mackay, D. G. (1981). The problem of rehearsal or mental practice. *Journal of Motor Behaviour, 13*, 274 –285.

Mackay, D. G. (1982). The problems of flexibility, fluency and speed-accuracy trade-off in skilled behaviour. *Psychological Review, 89*, 483–506.

Mazur, J., and Hastie, R. (1978). Learning as accumulation: A re-examination of the learning curve. *Psychological Bulletin, 85*, 1256–1274.

Neisser, U., Hirst, W., and Spelke, E. S. (1981). Limited capacity theories and the notion of automaticity: a reply to Lucas and Bub. *Journal of Experimental Psychology: General 110*, 499–500.

Newell, A., and Rosenbloom, P. S. (1981). Mechanisms of skill acquisition and the law of practice. In J. R. Anderson (Ed.). *Cognitive skills and their acquisition.* Hillsdale, NJ: Erlbaum.

Norman, D. A., and Shallice, T. (1980). *Attention to action: willed and automatic control of behaviour.* La Jolla, CA: Center for Human Information Processing Report 99.

Ornstein, R. E. (1972). *The psychology of consciousness.* San Francisco: Freeman.

Pew, R. W. (1966). Acquisition of hierarchical control over the temporal organisation of a skill. *Journal of Experimental Psychology, 71*, 764–771.

Pew, R. W. (1974). Human perceptual-motor performance. In B. H. Kantowitz (Ed.) *Human information processing.* Hillsdale, NJ: Erlbaum.

Poulton, E. C. (1957). On prediction in skilled movements. *Psychological Bulletin, 54,* 467–478.

Pylyshyn, Z. W. (1981). The imagery debate: analogue media versus tacit knowledge. *Psychological Review, 88,* 16–45.

Rabbitt, P. M. A. (1981). Sequential reactions. In D. H. Holding (Ed.) *Human skills.* Chichester: Wiley.

Richardson, A. (1967a, b). Mental practice: a review and discussion. Part I. *Research Quarterly, 38,* 95–107. Part 2. *Research Quarterly 38,* 263 –273.

Rumelhart, D. E., and Norman, D. A. (1982). Simulating a skilled typist: a study of skilled cognitive motor performance. *Cognitive Science, 6,* 1–36.

Schmidt, R. A. (1975). A schema theory of discrete motor skill learning. *Psychological Review, 82,* 225–260.

Schneider, W., and Eberts, R. (1980). *Consistency at multiple levels in sequential motor output processing.* Technical Report 80-4, Human Attention Research Laboratory, University of Illinois.

Schneider, W., and Fisk, A. D. (1982). Attention theory and mechanisms for skilled performances. In R. A. Magill (Ed.) *Memory and control of motor behavior.* Amsterdam: North Holland.

Shaffer, L. H. (1981). Performances of Chopin, Bach and Bartok: studies in motor programming. *Cognitive Psychology, 13,* 326–376.

Shiffrin, R. M., and Dumais, S. T. (1981). The development of automatism. In J. R. Anderson (Ed.) *Cognitive skills and their acquisition.* Hillsdale, NJ: Erlbaum.

Author Index

Page numbers in *italics* refer to bibliography.

Subject Index